W9-BGC-758

*Surviving Your Spouse's Chronic Illness*

# Surviving Your Spouse's Chronic Illness

## A COMPASSIONATE GUIDE

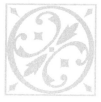

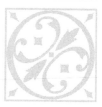

Chris McGonigle, Ph.D.

*An Owl Book*
HENRY HOLT AND COMPANY
NEW YORK

Henry Holt and Company, Inc.
*Publishers since 1866*
115 West 18th Street
New York, New York 10011

Henry Holt® is a registered
trademark of Henry Holt and Company, Inc.

Library of Congress Cataloging-in-Publication Data

McGonigle, Chris.
Surviving your spouse's chronic illness: a compassionate guide/
by Chris McGonigle.—1st ed.
p.    cm.
Includes index.
ISBN 0-8050-5573-8 (pbk.: alk. paper)
1. Chronically ill—Family relationships.    2. Chronically ill—Care.
3. Chronic diseases—Psychological aspects.    I. Title.
RC108.M39      1999                     98-23240
616'.044'019—dc21                        CIP

Henry Holt books are available for special promotions and
premiums. For details contact: Director, Special Markets.

First Edition 1999

Designed by Kate Nichols

Printed in the United States of America
All first editions are printed on acid-free paper. ∞

1    2    3    4    5    6    7    8    9    10

FOR DON, WHO BELIEVED IN ME

# Acknowledgments

To all the well spouses who made this book possible by sharing your most intimate thoughts and feelings, thank you. You are my heroes. My deep appreciation also to Stephanie Abarbanel, editor-at-large at *Family Circle*, who said, "Why don't you write it for us?"; Diana Finch, my agent, who patiently helped me shape an idea; Cynthia Vartan, the most skillful of editors; and all those who referred, explained, enlightened, and lent an encouraging word: Maggie Strong; Debbie Hayden; Tom Eastman; Don Crawford; Mary Lambert; Taryn Phillips-Quinn; Meg Lundstrom; Russ Cater; Sherrie Downing; Martha Vogt; Susan Brace; Pam Cavallo; Catherine Bryan; Kathy O'Connor; John Rolland, M.D.; Robert Shepard, M.D.; Pat Pasini; Charles Anderson, M.D.; Chadene Atkins; Catherine Shea; Kay Flinn; Carol McEvoy; Pat Still; Shevy Healey; Debra Borys; Randolph Schiffer, M.D.; Tom Campbell, M.D.; James Gormally; Laura Cooper. I'm grateful to my children, Megan McGonigle Gittings and Tim McGonigle, for their enthusiasm and encouragement, and to my parents, Jack and Elizabeth Caldwell, whose love has never failed me.

# Contents

*Surviving Your Spouse's Chronic Illness*

# Introduction

 "I wish he would die!" I sat on my parents' sofa and buried my face in my hands. They watched helplessly, having long since run out of words to comfort me. My husband had multiple sclerosis, and had been in a nursing home for five years. For what felt like the umpteen-millionth time, I wondered how I could go on watching him suffer. How I wanted it to be over, for him and for me.

I remember the devastation I felt when Don was diagnosed at age thirty-two. I was still young at twenty-nine, and though I loved him deeply, I knew that I might have a very long siege ahead. I went to counselors, who offered a sympathetic ear, but none of them had lived with a sick spouse. I found books about MS for Don that suggested techniques and diets and agencies that could make life easier. There was a local as well as a national MS support group.

But there was nothing for me, nothing that addressed the

emotional turmoil I felt as the wife of a man with a chronic illness. I looked in vain for books that told me someone else had walked where I was walking. *Hadn't anyone ever gone through this before?* I wondered. *Where were they? Why hadn't they written about it?* I felt unbearably lonely as I watched my friends, whose healthy husbands climbed career ladders and took their kids camping on weekends. I felt like I existed behind a plate glass barrier. I felt invisible.

Over the years, a few books on having a sick family member appeared, but they all focused on being a caregiver, which, to me, was the most manageable part of my life. These books seldom addressed how it felt to have a husband or wife come down with a serious illness. When they did, they sounded superficial and impossibly cheery. "Think of caregiving as a choice you have made," advised one. I was willing to concede that. I was still here, wasn't I? But no one in her right mind would choose to take care of someone twenty-four hours a day, day in, day out, for years. And years.

These books also lumped spouses in with other family members. But having a husband or wife become ill is very different from having a sick parent or child; so much more is at stake. You don't depend on your child for money or sex, two of the biggest sources of conflict in any marriage, whether the partners are sick or well. Maggie Strong's book *Mainstay*, appearing in 1988, was a watershed for well spouses. Finally, someone was talking honestly about one experience. The book called for well spouses to organize and help each other, and the Well Spouse Foundation was the result.

The notion that we might aspire to lives beyond that of full-time caregivers doesn't seem to occur to professionals. Numerous times as I was researching this book, I was assured that "there are plenty of books out there," only to be directed to the growing collection of caregiving books. The assumption that being a care-giver, and that alone, should provide all the satisfaction we need was both revealing and disheartening.

The well spouse experience is full of forbidden emotions. Reading the anonymous letters to the "Forum" section of the Well Spouse Foundation newsletter, *Mainstay*, I realized why the book I wanted for so many years didn't exist. In the face of soci-etal expectations that being a caregiver is completely fulfilling, it's too hard for spouses to admit their real feelings. I knew it was safe to tell my parents I wanted Don to die. They had seen me through the ordeal from the beginning, and they understood. But my friends wouldn't have understood. It's not acceptable to be angry with—to hate, on occasion—your sick husband or wife. It's not acceptable to resent the money that's spent on drugs and treatments and equipment. It's not acceptable to be repulsed by your mate's withering body. It's not acceptable, in other words, to talk about the reality of chronic illness in a marriage—what one wife called "the last closet."

Living with a loved one's illness is tragedy enough, but not being able to talk about it is a double tragedy. After every inter-view I did for this book, I mailed a copy of the transcript back to the interviewee to be checked for accuracy. I was often dismayed when it came back with the most honest statements sanitized, or accompanied by the request that I quote the statement anony-mously. "I'm sure it's hard for Larry too," one wife wrote in the margin of a passionate paragraph detailing how she hated some of her caregiving duties.

Yes, it's hard for Larry, as it is for all the ill members of our marriages. But it's hard for us too. And we make a bad situation worse when we can't share the truth about it.

A conspiracy of silence surrounds us because our reality dif-fers so dramatically from public perception. A magazine recently featured an article about Dana Reeve, whose husband, Christopher Reeve, star of the movie *Superman*, is paralyzed from the neck down from a horse-riding accident. The article was called "Woman of Steel." The title typifies the way the world wants to see us, as stronger than they, able to leap tall buildings at a single bound. But steel can be mummifying. When we begin to believe the myths that surround us, we're prevented from asking for help because we labor under the mistaken belief that other well spouses are coping better than we are, that we shouldn't need help. Reaching out for help is one of the hardest things we learn to do as well spouses. We need first of all to see it as a strength, not a weakness. I wish I had recognized this truth much earlier than I did. The people who came into our lives when I asked saved our lives.

According to a 1996 study by the Robert Wood Johnson Foundation, forty-one million people are "limited in their daily activities" by chronic illness. As the huge number of baby boomers age, this number will increase. Because antibiotics and other drugs keep people alive far longer than in the past, more couples are getting "slapped by the helping hand." ALS, or Lou Gehrig's disease, used to kill within a year or two. Yet I interviewed a beleaguered young wife whose husband is starting his seventh year with ALS. He's alive but has no quality of life. In the past five years, AIDS has been transformed from an acute to a chronic illness. Some forms of cancer have become chronic rather than acute. These "successes" represent the dark side of American medicine. Americans are living longer, but many have illnesses that limit their ability to really live—to ambulate, work, interact with their families, enjoy life. With no extended family to help shoulder the caregiving duties, as in the past, spouses do it all. The toll on these husbands and wives is inestimable.

Watching your husband or wife sicken is suffering like no other. It was an ordeal I lived for fifteen years, as my husband died slowly of MS. After his death in 1993, I wanted to write a book about the emotional and psychological aspects of the experience, because I knew how much a book would have helped me. I wanted, by sharing my own experiences and those of others, to reassure you that you aren't crazy, or selfish, or lustful, or deceitful, or plain bad. I wanted to find out what other spouses have thought and said and done and share it with you. I wanted to share my mistakes, in the hope that you can avoid them, and my insights in the hope that you can benefit from them. I've been sparing with "expert" advice. You and I are the experts.

Most of those interviewed for this book were willing to be identified by their full names. When someone requested anonymity, I changed details as well as names so that they weren't identifiable. With one exception, noted in the text, when a person is called by first and last names, the name is real. Single names are pseudonyms, but the words quoted were spoken by a real person.

If your spouse is newly diagnosed, you may find parts of this book hard to read. Remember that your spouse may never become as incapacitated as some of those here, and you may never find yourself in these circumstances. By interviewing more than forty spouses with widely varying temperaments, financial situations, and belief systems, whose husbands and wives have different illnesses and degrees of involvement, I've tried to offer a range of viewpoints, insights, and methods of coping. Knowing in advance what could happen can help prepare you if you encounter a similar obstacle in your own life. Knowledge is power.

Above all, I tried to keep in mind that you are, as I was, an ordinary person in an extraordinary situation. You're trying to fulfill a promise you made, yet find room for yourself within that commitment. You need to know that others have been here before you and survived. You need permission to get what you need, or, in the words of one wife, "to find the door," whatever that may mean to you. I hope this book helps.

# I. Diagnosis:
# Losing the Future

Diane Maxwell will never forget that morning in June 1976 when her husband, Jim, woke up unable to walk. The nightmare had begun the previous afternoon, when they had driven from their hometown of Polson, Montana, to the larger town of Missoula to see a neurologist recommended by their family doctor. The neurologist had leaned back in his chair and cocked his head at Jim, whose facial numbness was causing his left eye to droop. "You want to be sick, so you're sick," he said. He reached for a prescription pad and wrote out an order for Valium. "You should probably see a psychiatrist," he said disapprovingly.

The hour drive home in their new blue pickup was a blur for twenty-one-year-old Diane, who felt like her head was going to spin off, out the window, onto the pavement. *How can he be doing this to me?* she raged silently. *And why?* She loved him. After three years of marriage, she felt she knew intimately this big, soft man who could talk to a wall and get it to answer. Every furious thought was followed as quickly by a guilty one. *He's really sick,* another voice inside her head insisted. *You can't fake a drooping eye!* Round and round her thoughts boiled. *If I can see it, I must be crazy too,* she concluded.

Diane was fixing breakfast the next morning when she heard Jim's strangled call for help. In the hallway, she was horrified to see him trying to crawl to her on his hands and knees. "I can't walk," he croaked. Awkwardly, she pulled on his shorts and T-shirt and half-dragged, half-carried him to the truck. Throwing his shoes in the back of the truck, she told him grimly, "We're going back to the doctor, and we're not leaving till we get some answers."

As she sat in the small waiting room while Jim underwent laboratory tests, Diane couldn't stop the memories that flooded past. After their marriage, she and Jim had bought a refrigeration repair business in the tiny, scenic town on the shores of Flathead Lake. The land they planned to build a house on was covered with wildflowers and ponderosa pine. The business was flourishing, and Diane hoped to be pregnant soon. But the doctor's words to her that afternoon changed all that. They were about Jim, and they were bad. "I think he has MS."

Diane's first thoughts were not for Jim, but for herself. She was afraid she was going to start screaming in front of everybody. *Maybe they'll have to tie me down, drag me off,* she thought.

Diane didn't know much about MS, but she knew from the TV ads that it was "the silent crippler of young adults." The doctor thought Jim was too distraught to hear the news, and Diane agreed. Her twenty-eight-year-old husband had had a difficult childhood, and was still dealing with the horrors of Vietnam. The doctor scheduled a CAT scan in Seattle, where Jim's cousins distracted them with trips to the beach and the Space Needle and allowed Jim to regain some equilibrium. True to her word, Diane kept the ugly secret from Jim, sneaking out of bed in the middle of the night to call her sister and cry. Within a week they were back in the doctor's office. The CAT scan had ruled out a brain tumor, allowing the doctor to make a diagnosis by elimination. Now Jim knew, too.

Whether the news comes suddenly or slowly, the diagnosis of serious illness obliterates the peaceful path a couple has been walking. The first symptoms of Alzheimer's disease throw a spouse into a murky netherworld where everything looks the same but different. Bill Hill's seventy-year-old wife, Peggy, began to complain that she couldn't find things, that "someone was taking things" from her. Exasperated, Bill helped her search the drawers of her dresser, until it dawned on him that she was moving things around herself. Peggy's lack of affection troubled him too. Bill had been a career U.S. Marine Corps officer, and they were always extra affectionate when he was home, trying to make up for lost time. Now Peggy began to turn away. Still capable of understanding that she was behaving strangely, she agreed to a neurological examination. Bill got the diagnosis piecemeal. "The average physician doesn't want to put himself on the spot diagnosing Alzheimer's," says Bill. "And they may have been cautious around her." Instead, Peggy's doctor gave him the report of her neurological workup. Determined, Bill read it through twice before his eyes snagged on the phrase "atrophy of the cortical section of the brain." After the doctor handed him pamphlets on Alzheimer's, he knew. Bill liked the fact that the doctors gave him the devastating news gently. "They didn't just drop it on me."

Sometimes the diagnosis comes as a relief, at least for a while. Jim Russell's wife, Hannah, was forty-one when, out of the blue, her right leg began to drag. Avid walkers, the Russells frequently took five-mile treks into the Connecticut countryside. One warm Memorial Day, they walked downtown for the big parade, with fire engines and Cub Scouts and clowns. Or rather, Jim walked. Hannah suddenly couldn't. "What's wrong?" Jim asked impatiently. "The parade's already started." Hannah was baffled. "I don't know," she replied. "It just . . ." she tried to explain the odd sensation of a limb suddenly gone missing ". . . doesn't work." Every time he turned around, she was farther behind. Jim didn't think Hannah was the type to pretend, but he couldn't account for her problems any other way. *What kind of game is she playing?* he fumed to himself. Angrily, he picked her up and carried her to the curb, where they watched the parade in silence.

Hannah immediately reported to their family doctor, who recommended physical therapy. Over the next few weeks, Hannah's right leg continued to give out, especially in the afternoons when she was tired. Jim, who had fallen in love with her midwestern practicality and common sense, began to wonder how he had misread her character so completely. What kind of woman had he married, who would fake something like this? Was she mentally unstable? He examined her leg for signs of redness or swelling, but there were none, nor had she injured herself in any way. How else to explain this unless it was all in her head?

After weeks of whirlpool baths and exercises produced no results, the doctor sent Hannah to a neurologist. Jim was pouring drinks for friends the evening Hannah returned from her hospital tests. "They think I have MS," she said. *Thank God,* Jim thought. *It's not a mystery anymore.* He had never heard of MS, but at least it was something real. They even had a name for it! If they could name it, they must be able to cure it, he thought. *She won't be heading to the insane asylum and taking me with her.*

At last, after weeks of uncertainty, there was something he could do: find out about MS. He visited several libraries, collecting articles and books and photocopying anything he wanted to read later. When he sat down to read, he felt as though he had closed the door on one kind of hell and entered a new one. His horror and shock grew with each word. There were no treatments that helped and certainly no cure.

His world went dark. He and Hannah had been married four years, but he still thought of them as newlyweds. They both had good jobs, and had just bought a house on two wooded acres. The future seemed limitless. Now he searched Hannah's green eyes as if the answers lay somewhere inside them, and couldn't stop crying. There was no one and nothing to blame; the books were clear at least on that point. In the evening, he took a bottle of Jack Daniel's and sat in front of the TV, drinking until the pain receded. It became his daily routine.

My husband, Don, came home from a fishing trip one day in the summer of 1978 complaining that, as he was tramping through deep brush on the creek bank, he couldn't feel his legs for a few minutes. I looked at him, hot and sweaty but otherwise whole and sound and walking up the steps perfectly now, and put the comment out of my mind. He decided he was out of shape and began to get up before work and go jogging. Within a few days he told me that when he tried to run, he fell. I remembered the time two years earlier, when I was pregnant with Tim, that his forearms had gone numb for a few days. A little alarm bell began to ring in my brain. I had two aunts with MS, two of my mother's sisters. One had problems with double vision, but nothing else. The other had been in a nursing home, helpless, for several years. With a jolt of pure terror, I remembered that her MS had started with problems walking. I was teaching English at a local college, and one evening after class I went to the library and read up on MS. In one case I read about, a man's hand went numb for a few hours once a year, interfering with his golf game. In another case, a young woman died within months. I spiraled dizzily between the certainty that Don was going to be fine, that his difficulties walking were like the man's numb hand, minor and fleeting, and the equally strong certainty that he had only months to live. Don visited our family doctor, who scheduled an appointment with a neurologist for a myelogram. Dr. Shepard must have suspected MS, but I was the one who first mentioned it. His response was curious. "I wouldn't have brought it up if you hadn't," he said. He wasn't ready to even admit out loud that it might be what Don had. Neither was the neurologist, who scrawled at the bottom of his notes that Don had "spasticity of lower legs, etiology unknown." We returned home, Don with a nagging spinal headache, to await the next symptom.

I had never had anxiety attacks, but I got them now, with terrifying intensity. At times I couldn't perform the smallest task, such as getting dressed, fixing breakfast, even pushing myself out of bed. What difference did any of it make, I wondered, when my thirty-two-year-old husband could be dying? What would this illness do to him, our five-year-old marriage, and our two small children? Don's ability to continue with his life as if nothing had happened added to my sense of unreality. I, too, wondered who was crazy, him or me? It was the only time in my life I've ever taken tranquilizers.

That crazy period of my life could have been shortened if there had been tests that diagnosed MS—not just ruled out other things, but ruled in MS. Some illnesses are easier to diagnose than others; Parkinson's victims have a characteristic stoic expression that, to medical professionals, gives them away. One wife recalls the doctor telling her, "I could tell your husband had Parkinson's from watching him in the waiting room." Fortunately, MS now can be diagnosed with an MRI scan, but a baffled patient is still at the mercy of the family doctor, who, not recognizing the signs of neurological disease, may prescribe tranquilizers instead of referring him or her to a neurologist. Lucky the couple who finds themselves in front of a physician who makes similar diagnoses all the time, because they will be spared the hell of waiting for the other shoe to drop. The diagnosis of incurable disease, as Bill Hill noted of Alzheimer's, is one that physicians are reluctant to make. No one wants to be the bearer of bad news, and doctors are human like the rest of us. Since several of these hopeless illnesses are neurological—Alzheimer's, Parkinson's, ALS, MS—with symptoms that come and go, diagnosing them is often a deadly earnest game of hide-and-seek.

The doctors dangled tantalizing carrots before Don and me. He might have "post-polio syndrome," the aftereffects of the polio he had as a child, or it might be a lack of vitamin B. It could even be Guillain-Barré syndrome, a serious but usually reversible paralysis.

We waited an endless year, with Don faithfully taking vitamins and both of us hoping against hope that one day he would awaken and be completely normal. Then he began to have a sort of electric-shock sensation down his spine when he bent his head forward. This symptom, called Lehrmitte's Sign, was considered proof of MS, as the neurologist told us at the end of that year. By then, he also had begun to have problems urinating, and I realized that whatever was affecting the walking nerves was affecting another site too. So, in spite of the expensive, painful tests, and the trips to other towns, and dealing with an arrogant specialist who spoke only neurological-ese, Don and I were the ones who made the diagnosis. His walking and balance were not going to get better, because he had MS. "Why is this happening?" I begged Don as we held each other at night. I couldn't accept that my big, handsome husband, the man I believed I would grow old with, might die before me. "I don't know, Chrissie," he replied, clutching me tighter.

Words can't describe the violence of a serious diagnosis. All the plans, dreams, and hopes we shared with our partner are suddenly torn away. We're robbed of something infinitely precious: the future we planned on with a beloved husband or wife. The grief feels overwhelming and unremitting, hitting again and again in unexpected ways. Just as you think you're starting to make peace with this new reality, something reminds you, and you're drowning, yet again, in grief. One shimmering summer day we took a drive, and catching sight of a sign that said "Pony Rides," we stopped. As Megan, age five, and Tim, age two, clamored to be led around on the pony, Don fiddled with the camera in his lap. "I'll just take some pictures," he said, and I realized he wasn't up to walking that day. *What's wrong with this picture?* I thought. Young family, cute kids, perfect summer day, a winsome pony peering out from under his bushy mane. Except the handsome young husband has a dreadful disease. I wanted to lie down in the meadow and go to sleep until the nightmare was over.

To complicate things, grief is a hydra-headed monster, with faces of numbness, shock, anger, denial, and blame. Denial, writes Shelley Taylor in *Positive Illusions: Creative Self-Deception and the Healthy Mind*, is "one of the most primitive of human defenses." According to Elisabeth Kubler-Ross's widely regarded paradigm of the grief process, denial is often our first response to bad news. The police must be mistaken, the tests must be wrong, the illness is really just a vitamin deficiency. Denial, which I'll discuss in more detail in the next chapter, is a reflex. It is the psychological equivalent of putting your hands out to break a fall. It provides a merciful cushion between us and misfortune, a way to keep tragic events from overwhelming us psychologically. Under normal circumstances, denial abates so that we can absorb the new reality a little at a time. Like the numbness that surrounds a flesh wound, it eases us into accepting the unacceptable—and with illnesses that are completely unacceptable, there is lots of denial, by both the victims and their family members. Everything in us strives to keep things the same, to bar this unwelcome intruder from the door, to stay normal just a little bit longer.

Particularly at first, the denial mechanism can be amazingly strong. With their two sons nearly grown, Hilde and Hank had just taken in two foster daughters, ages three and five, from an abusive home. The decision had been a lengthy and difficult one for them. Now Hilde looked at her husband, close to death from a car accident, and thought, against all reason, "He'll be all right soon."

"This is how my mind worked," she says wonderingly. "I thought, 'it's OK that he looks like this, that he's had this operation and he can barely breathe, as long as he's fine by November.'" He had to be all right by then, because they had a doctor's appointment for the girls. "I thought, you can lie here and be like this as long as you want, but by the nineteenth of November, we have to be in Salt Lake City."

Kas Enger, whose husband, Ken, has had MS for fifteen years, says, "There have been times when I've wanted to say, 'Would you just stop being sick now? Just cut it out!' Even though you know that's not logical, everything in your being just wants him to go back to the way he was. I felt like a little kid that stiffens up and throws a tantrum when she doesn't get her way."

When it's the sick one who's denying, he often has no trouble convincing a partner, who desperately wants to believe it's something else, too. Bette Allbright's husband, Jim, was certain that he didn't have MS. He didn't know what he did have, just something else that had a cure. After years of his trying to persuade her, she got exasperated. "I had enough doubt and hope that it worked for a while," she admits. "But I finally told him to stop brainwashing me." Another woman traveled to various medical centers throughout the United States, submitting to grueling myelograms again and again, hoping that her diagnosis eventually would be something other than MS.

As if our own reactions weren't enough to deal with, we have to deal with our spouse's reactions too. Couples may feel as if they've received two separate diagnoses, and in a way they have. Grief separates even the most compatible partners because, simply put, it's pain—pain that we must work through alone before we can reach out to our partners. The news of a spouse's serious illness changes perception. We suddenly realize that we, too, are mortal, subject to the same misfortunes as this person whose life is so inextricably entwined with ours. If this catastrophe can happen to them, something equally fearsome can happen to us too. Suddenly, with no warning, we're staring death in the face. At a time when we need each other the most, we're least able to reach out for each other.

Typically, men stay in the "alone" stage longer. For them, grief is humiliating because they're supposed to know how to handle crises; they feel weak if they confess their own fear and sadness and confusion. The need to withdraw is a primitive, instinctive one, one we share with animals. After we assess our wounds and realize they aren't fatal, we're ready to rejoin the herd.

However, a husband's silence can make a wife feel more isolated than ever, when what she needs is to talk about what's happening to them. If she begs him to share his feelings, he may retreat even further, feeling as if, after all he's lost, someone wants something more from him. If she tries to remind him that his illness affects her, too, she may meet with rejection. I remember Don saying to me, "This isn't happening to you," a devastating remark when I was seeing my own life go down the toilet too. I wanted to scream, "I'm your wife! It *is* happening to me!"

Logically, of course, he was right. It was his legs that wouldn't always support him, his hands that sometimes let a glass slip to the floor and shatter, his eyes that sometimes misread the colors of traffic lights. He was experiencing a betrayal of the most fundamental kind. Only after he had had time to absorb his own emotions did he allow me in.

Some partners want to "be strong" for the other, as Diane Maxwell did, but this course of action can be unbearably isolating, as she discovered. We hold back our own distress because we don't want to burden our partners further, when it may be reassuring to discover we're experiencing similar feelings.

Some spouses want to fix the hurt, and, like Jim Russell, feel frustrated and helpless when they find out there are no fixes. Discovering this hard fact brings yet another kind of isolation. After all, so many illnesses, in our great United States, are fixable. It's no exaggeration to say that we live in an age of miracles, where no medical feat seems beyond our reach, and new marvels are reported daily in the media. A spouse whose partner has contracted something incurable feels disoriented, as if, somehow, he's fallen into a time warp. As one man said of his wife's incurable diagnosis, "I thought of it as King Arthur's Castle. A gate came down, separating us from the rest of the world."

When Don got MS in 1978, I had that walled-off sensation, too, as if I lived among the lepers and paralytics of the Bible. As far as devastating neurological diseases, medical research had virtually stood still. By the time Don died fifteen years later, that was still true. It was no comfort to hear Don's neurologist tell us that the lack of knowledge wasn't due to a lack of research. "MS has just been a real rascal to pin down," he said.

Not only did medicine not have a cure for this illness, but no one had any idea of what caused it or how it might unfold. "My crystal ball is a bowling ball," a doctor admitted to me once with refreshing candor, and his remark pretty much sums up what is known about chronic illness. In those early weeks after Don's diagnosis, despite literature from the MS Society assuring us that MS was not considered life-threatening, I grieved my husband's death. Sometimes, in fact, I mourned him so completely that when he walked in the door after work, I felt a shock, as though he had come back from the dead.

Diagnosis introduces the first of many such "ambiguous losses." Although the future with the spouse may be gone, he or she is still here. The illness is probably not too bad yet, and maybe it will never get too bad. How much grief is called for at this stage? we wonder. We're afraid we're being hysterical, overreacting, if we feel overcome with sadness, especially if our partners are carrying on stoically. I had to anticipate the worst outcome, my husband's death, in order to get to the other side and to be able to appreciate all the things he still could do. Others may be able to postpone the worst of their grief until the illness worsens. There's no right or wrong way to get through this difficult time.

The uncertainty of what the future holds denies us the luxury of grieving fully. Norma Imber knows. Love was lovelier the second time around for Norma, whose first husband died of a heart attack at age thirty-eight. Richard had been somewhat cold and rigid, but Robert, an interior decorator, was his total opposite. "His love was so strong that if I was in the bedroom, and he was in the living room, I could feel those waves. So that tells you," she says. Robert was sixty-five when he had a severe stroke that left him brain damaged and unable to walk. Although her first husband's death was a terrible shock, at least it was final. "In my experience, that's the way to go," she says. "Not this chronic illness. It just seems like there's no light at the end of the tunnel."

Psychologists say that the flip side of depression is anxiety, which, in the absence of a definite diagnosis, can paint terrifying pictures. Psychologist Daniel Goleman has described anxiety as "cognitive static," and that's exactly what it feels like, a noisy radio with the "off" button missing. The radio plays loudest during those long delays when the doctors prescribe tranquilizers, or physical therapy, or tests that prove inconclusive. Because getting a diagnosis often involves anguishing delays, we have periods of time without any answers, and our imaginations run wild. As Diane Maxwell and Jim Russell found, it's easy to think one of you is crazy, and you have times when you're convinced you both are.

For each couple, the losses are staggering. Diane Maxwell and her husband were starting a new business and trying to start a family. Bill and Peggy Hill, with both of their sons launched, were starting to enjoy Bill's being home—no more long separations courtesy of the U.S. Marine Corps. Jim and Hannah Russell had good jobs and were consulting a fertility specialist. Hilde and Hank planned to provide a loving home for two damaged children. Norma and Robert Imber were savoring each moment of a blissful second marriage and were planning to travel, now that Robert had retired. Another couple, Mark and Bonnie Johannes, had gotten some marriage counseling and their relationship "was becoming really great," according to Mark. Bonnie's diagnosis of MS was a macabre gift, arriving four days before their ninth anniversary. It's no wonder that the grief which results from such losses can feel too big to resolve.

Catastrophe on this scale reminds us of the insignificance of individual human life in a vast, uncaring universe. In an effort to regain some control, we grope for reasons and causes. We seize on explanations, look for someone or something to blame, no matter how illogical. I couldn't help wondering if Don's polio had led to this second neurological illness twenty-five years later, although there was no medical research that even suggested such a thing. Or wondering if maybe his mother, a nurse, had given him too many antibiotics as a child and confused his immune system, which now couldn't tell his own nerve tissue from a bacterium, and so was attacking it. I was so irrationally furious with his father one afternoon that I could barely look at him. *It's all your fault!* I thought. *It's your fault and Margaret's fault, because you had him for the first twenty-six years of his life! You sold me damaged goods!* I couldn't say how or why it was their fault, I just knew it was. The blaming was one more example of the craziness of my grief. No explanation seemed too absurd.

Laura's husband was recuperating from the myelogram that had just diagnosed his ALS when he was served with an arrest warrant for embezzlement. For her, his trouble with the law was worse than the illness. She was humiliated by the knowledge that her small community saw her husband, Marv, as a thief and a liar. She describes him as "a man with lots of shadows," and wonders if he didn't pick out his own disease "as a respectable way out." The question still haunts her, now that he is dead. Our inability to find reasons mocks our human need to know why.

Life after diagnosis alternates between feeling totally out of control and suffocatingly small. My dreams echoed with the sound of iron gates slamming closed. In one particularly vivid dream, Don had fallen on his back on a steep hillside, and I was holding on to his hands from above, trying to pull him up. He was too heavy for me to pull him to safety, but I couldn't let go either. I still remember the sweaty desperation of that dream, the need to save him exactly proportionate to the hopelessness of the situation. How, I wondered, could the enormous love I felt for him feel like such a trap? The dream had captured perfectly the dilemma I was in, then and for many years to come.

"Run," my instincts screamed. I dreamed of packing the car and the children and heading out, I didn't know where, just someplace safe, and starting over with a new, healthy husband— no one I knew, just someone untainted. I looked around at the healthy young men in my English classes and wondered why I couldn't be married to one of them instead. Why had Don been singled out for this curse?

Jane Dibert's sixty-year-old husband, Bill, had quadruple bypass surgery, and now they live with his chronic angina and the imminent possibility of another heart attack. After Bill came home from the hospital, Jane felt panicky. "It was an overwhelming feeling of not wanting to be in that time and place," she says. She recognized that such feelings were probably normal, and was able to reassure herself that she was not a bad person to have them. A high school biology teacher, Jane found that returning to the classroom after Christmas vacation was all the escape she needed; otherwise, she believes, she would have had to find another way to get out of the house each day, at least for a while.

Those of us who are reeling at the thought that the healthy person we married is not healthy, may wonder how couples can marry knowing one of them has a chronic illness. We wonder why they don't run while they have a chance.

Linda Anderson knew that the young man she had met at church had MS, but that didn't stop her from falling in love. She didn't know anyone who had MS, and didn't want to read about it. She thought they would be lucky, and Steve thought so, too. He had six good years before his health began to slip. Reflecting on his death at age forty-four, Linda sighs, "Had I known at the beginning what we were facing, I probably wouldn't have married him." She believes they had a good marriage, in spite of his illness. "I wouldn't want that knowledge in advance, but looking back, everything that's come from it, I don't regret any of my decisions."

For Linda, an illness that hadn't unsheathed its claws yet was still a pussycat in the corner, as it was for nineteen-year-old Gaelene Farrell, who met her husband, Wayne, at Yellowstone

National Park, where they were seasonal workers. Unlike Linda Anderson, Gaelene knew what she could be getting into. Wayne had diabetes, which had killed her grandmother. "She was supposed to take insulin shots, but hated needles," Gaelene said. "She ate everything she wanted, and the way I came to see it, she was killing herself."

For Gaelene, then, diabetes seemed to be a disease one could control. Wayne took care of himself; her grandmother hadn't. "I figured he was never going to end up the way my grandma had," she says. "He wasn't sick, had no pain anywhere, no trouble with his eyes." Her grandfather wasn't happy about her decision to marry Wayne. "Grandpa didn't like Wayne, and now I think maybe his illness was part of the reason," she says.

All couples, married yet or not, with a serious diagnosis, share things in common. We all tend, in this early stage, to indulge in magical thinking and to believe we have more control over the outcome of the illness than is really the case—but that's not necessarily bad. Don took vitamins, and we tried a gluten-free diet. With illnesses like MS, where nothing had been proven to help, these things helped us feel we had some control. Although they had no effect on the outcome of Don's illness, the emotional effect was helpful, because we felt we were banding together against a common enemy. For a while, we believed we could control the MS through sheer force of will, and keep it at bay with the strength of our love, which helped us weather that post-diagnosis trauma.

Most professionals advise learning as much as you can about the illness. Knowing what to expect can save you from making snap decisions. But we all have different readiness thresholds for this information, and that must be respected, too. I have always felt that forewarned is forearmed, and sought out as much information as I could. Then, I consulted with our doctor about my husband's case. Keep in mind, too, that illness takes very different courses in different people. Your spouse may never become as incapacitated as the literature describes. Your husband or wife may be among the lucky few who have light cases, or for whom a new drug prevents the development of serious complications.

Couples who already know a diagnosis before marriage are at least spared the initial shock and the crazy, unbalanced time that follows it. This post-diagnosis chaos is the first of many transitions a couple negotiates over the course of a chronic illness. The turmoil created by a diagnosis may actually be useful, in that it makes possible a new life that accommodates the illness. That transition takes time, however, and the interim can feel like tumbling out a window at sixty miles an hour.

In crises, people revert to methods of comfort that have worked in the past, so if a mate has always gone off by himself to digest bad news, expect him to do it now and be patient. Trust your own instincts to tell you when he's been gone too long. Then you might ask him how he's doing with the news, and tell him how you're doing with it. Even though both of you are in pain, you can still reach out a hand to each other. A terrified partner needs our reassurance. "She was afraid I might leave," says Bill Hill of his wife after they learned her Alzheimer's diagnosis. "I said, 'I'm not leaving. I'm taking care of you.'" If you're married to someone who wants to talk, you can arrange times and places to do that. Your future happiness may depend on it. Recognize that you aren't feeling anything that millions of others haven't felt in this stressful time. Panic, longing to escape, blaming, anger at your spouse, terror, enormous grief—these emotions are all part of getting the news. As one wife said, "We beat ourselves up for normal feelings. This is one of those journeys you have to go through to understand."

With a serious diagnosis, the prism through which we look at life begins to change, and it must. With the future a gaping hole, we learn to put our eyes on what's in front of us in order to retain some sense of control. "One day at a time" was never as fitting as it is for those absorbing a serious diagnosis. With the awareness of life's fragility comes the recognition of how precious each moment is. We learn to savor that delicious piece of pie in front of us, the magazine on our laps, the sun on our shoulders, and say, *I don't know what's coming, but for now, I'm all right.*

Be assured that life, although it will never be normal again, will normalize. Daily life has a reassuring pull that we can't resist for long. There are meals to be cooked, babies to be diapered, sunsets to be watched. As life settles back into a routine, the quotidian seems precious as never before. You may not be able to control the future, but you have the here and now. Tell yourself you will deal with the next crisis when it comes, and trust yourself that you will.

# 2. Denial: "You Always Think You Have Time"

Whenever I hear that song about Cleopatra, Queen of Denial, I have to smile, because when it came to his MS, Don was the king. Denial has gotten a bad name in recent years, but looking back on Don's determination to ignore his increasing weakness and fatigue and plod doggedly on, I sometimes wonder if it isn't another name for courage. Denial, that dirty word, enabled him to function much longer than someone more "in touch with reality." I remember the astonishment on his doctor's face when she and I met privately after he had spent a week in her rehab unit. "He has an incredible ability to just overlook things that would stop me cold," she said.

The experience of chronic illness is filled with paradoxes, and denial is one of them. While it can play a positive part in coping with illness, both for us and for our partners, it can also be a continual sore spot. The worst thing about denial is the isolation it brings, both the physical isolation that comes when a partner refuses to use equipment that keeps him mobile, and the emotional isolation that comes because the wall of denial doesn't allow honest communication about the illness. Couples often differ dramatically about how an illness should be treated, or whether it should be treated at all. If to one of them it doesn't exist, why treat it? We find ourselves wanting desperately to see our partners as they see themselves: capable, in control, able to do everything they've done in the past, "their old selves." But allowing ourselves to be seduced against our better judgment can be fraught with danger, as some of the spouses in this chapter discovered.

The chronically ill are often reluctant to use any kind of adaptive equipment because it labels them as disabled. One wife insisted that she'd rather people thought she was drunk than that she had MS, a telling comment on the relative social acceptance of one condition compared to the other. Meantime, well spouses have nightmares about something happening that will take much more than a piece of equipment to put right. I was only too aware that if Don fell and broke his leg because he was too proud to use a walker, I would be the one who would be the day and night nurse until he recovered. We live in constant fear that a partner's stubbornness is going to do us in, in large ways and small.

In our culture, where people define themselves in terms of their profession, those with disabilities are stigmatized. Ours is a culture that idolizes youth and fitness, and disability is seen as a lack of character, a personal failing—something to be ashamed of. "I'd rather be dead than disabled" is a statement couples can expect to hear sooner or later. The roots of Yankee self-reliance and Calvinistic determinism run deep, and if you're not fixable, it's somehow your fault. Witness the ongoing controversy over terminology. The disabled reject terms like "handicapped" in favor of "handi-capable," and "disabled" for "differently abled." They may resent being called a "victim," or a "sufferer," who is

"confined to a wheelchair," words that, to them, describe limitations rather than abilities. The vehemence with which these
terms are rejected and the persistence of the debate speak volumes about our subtle but pervasive attitudes toward the handicapped. Don and I learned that we ignored these at our peril.

With its front and back steps, narrow hallways, and small
bathroom, the house we were living in soon became an obstacle
course for Don. When his uncle presented us with a check for a
down payment for a new house, we began looking at options.
Building would give us the chance to design a barrier-free house
from the ground up, rather than trying to make someone else's
house accessible, and having to work their avocado bathroom fix-
tures and burnt orange carpet into the bargain. We bought a piece
of land in an attractive neighborhood and signed up a contractor.
Not wanting to take chances, we decided to go ahead and sell our
house, rather than end up with two mortgage payments. Don told
me I had to go alone to meetings at the bank. "When they see me
in this chair, they'll start asking questions," he said. "I don't want
to give them a chance to refuse us." I did this with some trepida-
tion; it was the first time I had ever had to negotiate a big bank
loan, and my first lesson in having to become two people. More
fun was in store. With all Don's energy devoted to working an
eight-hour day, it also fell to me to find us a rental.

The problem was, there weren't any. Rentals of any kind were
scarce, but those with no stairs were virtually nonexistent. Anything with a split entry was automatically out, as were mobile
homes, which usually had steps up to the doors; and older homes
usually had bedrooms and bathrooms upstairs. I was shocked at
how having a family member unable to walk narrowed our housing choices. Finally, I thought I had located the perfect house, with
no steps, bedrooms and bath on the first floor, and a driveway
right beside the back door. When I called the owner, I innocently

told him we were building a house for my disabled husband, who was in a wheelchair, and we needed somewhere to live temporarily. "I couldn't rent to you then," he said bluntly. "You wouldn't be able to keep the yard up." I put down the phone, dumbfounded. This man thought it was perfectly all right to discriminate against handicapped people—he hadn't even bothered to make up a lie. Furious, I thought about calling the Human Rights Commission and filing a complaint. Then I remembered that we had to be out of our house in a few days, at which time we would be homeless, and put down the phone. *This is how it feels to be a minority*, I thought.

More housing-related troubles awaited. I was still unpacking boxes in the one-level apartment I finally found for us when the phone rang. It was the principal at Four Georgians School, calling to tell me that since we had moved out of his area, we had to move the kids to a different school. I protested. School had just started for the year; Tim was only a kindergartner, a tender new shoot in the school system. Our new house was in the Four Georgians area, and we'd be moving there in a few months. Why uproot the kids? It was adding insult to injury. I had scoured the town for an accessible house in the old neighborhood, and because I couldn't find one, the kids were being kicked out of their school. After a few months of letter-writing and bureaucratic conferring, they were allowed to stay put.

By February the new, frame one-story ranch house was ready. It had an open living and dining area, a big roll-in shower, wide hallways and doorways, and a ramp from the driveway into the back door. Don had to be at the closing to sign papers, but by then it was too late for the bank to refuse us a loan. The paperwork flowed smoothly. That night, in our spacious new living room, we breathed a sigh of relief. We were delighted with our new home, but I had an uneasy new knowledge of how completely Don's illness cut us off from the herd. It was the sheep and the goats all over again, and we had definitely ended up with the goats.

No wonder people with chronic illness hate to be seen using handicap equipment. They know and we know that these aids brand them in screaming neon colors as disabled, with all the preconceptions that calls up.

Don fought tooth and nail not to use a walker. He accepted a cane fairly readily, partly because of the "country squire" image that went along with it, and partly because it was fairly innocuous. Canadian crutches and walkers and wheelchairs, on the other hand, were things old people used, not young men in their prime. He feared people would see him as an illness, when he thought of himself as a functioning father, husband, and employee. "I don't make a very good poster boy," he'd say ruefully when I'd suggest renting or buying a piece of equipment.

I was torn. I wanted him to keep his muscles strong, and not depend on anything mechanical to do the work for them. I had to admire his independence, but it seemed way too early in the game to become a recluse. Was he being selfish for wanting to fight the MS his way, or was I being selfish for wanting to keep him part of the family? I couldn't decide. On Mother's Day his parents were coming to town and wanted to take us out to dinner. Visiting with Margaret and Ed was something I looked forward to, and when Don said, "I don't think I'm going to go, my legs are too weak today," I was disappointed and angry. "Can't we ever plan for these things?" I erupted. "You've known they were coming all week!" When he agreed to let me rent a wheelchair for him, I felt guilty, as if I was collaborating with the enemy. On the other hand, the disease was already taking so much away from us. I wasn't ready to hand over my husband. And with equipment so readily available, I couldn't understand how he could choose isolation rather than be with us.

He had to come to these decisions in his own time, and sometimes it took a crisis to convince him. I learned to keep one part of my brain on alert when he was in the house, listening for the sound of disaster. More than once, I was jolted into heart-pounding terror by the sound of a loud thump somewhere in the house, and I'd run, trying not to crash into anything myself, toward the source. As soon as he caught sight of my stricken face, he'd reassure me. "I'm all right, I'm all right," he'd say, and, incredibly, he always was. After we'd done an assessment and found that nothing was broken or spurting blood, we'd set about the task of getting him up off the floor. We became ingenious at getting his two-hundred-pound frame back in a sitting position. His upper body was still strong, so with me directing, Don suggesting, and the kids fetching the necessary items, we rolled him onto throw rugs and pulled him across the floor to a bed, where he could get into a kneeling position. Then we could slide the wheelchair under him. Once we used the kids' plastic sled, and one time it was their wagon. Over the years, the house's woodwork and plaster and linoleum bore the history of his sudden encounters with them. Once he grabbed at a dowel I had stuck into a plant to prop it up, and ended up in a heap of potting soil and crushed leaves.

One husband described these stages of denial and eventual acceptance as the "lowlights" of his wife's MS. "At the end of each of these stages, from a cane, to Canadian crutches, to a walker, leading to the wheelchair," he says, "she fell frequently, fighting her balance all the way and denying that she needed more assistance until eventually it became obvious even to her that she had to change." As much as we fret and hover, we can't force these changes on a partner, even when it's clearly for their own safety. "I get frustrated with him," says Diane Maxwell of her husband Jim's refusal to use a walker. "But I notice he drags his left foot more and more. It's only a matter of time." Frustration is the mildest emotion we feel; it's hard not to be livid when a preventable accident happens.

Kas Enger says, "Anything new, Ken resists." When they walked together, he used a cane but also leaned on her shoulder for balance. "I would just ache the next day," she says. "I told somebody I didn't realize it took so many muscles to go slowly. But it really did. So I finally talked him into the electric cart."

Sometimes trying to argue with a spouse causes physical distress that seems worse than the denial. Carly's husband, Mike, has had scleroderma for eight years, which has led to ARDS, acute respiratory distress syndrome. According to Carly, Mike has always had lots of denial. "He needed a chair to go up and down the stairs, and he was very, very resistant," she says. Mike liked to stay up late, so Carly would go to bed, only to be awakened night after night because Mike couldn't climb the stairs and needed her help. She knew she could order an automatic chair for the stairs, but she was afraid that Mike, in a fit of temper, would try to rip the chair out and then hyperventilate, which would lead to an attack of ARDS. So Carly went along month after month, afraid to rock the boat. Her growing exhaustion made her realize she needed to stand up to him. She ordered the chair and told him that if he had a fit, he would only harm himself. "I used to proclaim things way in advance," she says, "instead of just taking action and doing it. That was wrong."

Donna Keefe, age forty-three, faced a similar situation but came to a different decision. Her husband, Pat, age forty-seven, has chronic pancreatitis, and was so ill at one time he underwent a Whipple procedure, a last-ditch operation to reroute his entire gastrointestinal tract. The Whipple is so drastic, few survive it. Pat's doctor has forbidden him to drink, but Donna knows he drinks wine with his buddies, and she worries. "Wine is alcohol, too, and I don't think he should drink any," she says. But she has decided not to fight with him about it. Pat cannot work anymore, and so few things give him pleasure, Donna realizes. Besides, the stress of an argument causes him physical pain. "He'll just double over, and it makes his health a whole lot worse," she says. His drinking seems the lesser of two evils.

For Polly and Chuck, arguments about food poisoned their marriage. Even when they married, Polly was a hefty 160 pounds, but as she became more and more incapacitated by rheumatoid arthritis, her weight climbed. Deprived of activities that used to give her pleasure, she increasingly turned to food. As she gained weight, Chuck found it more and more difficult to lift her into and out of her wheelchair. This was both a physical and emotional strain for him. Transferring his wife gave them an opportunity for a "transfer hug," a time for intimacy that would be lost if they had to hire home health care workers. He felt that if Polly lost weight, she might regain some of her lost independence, and allow him to keep transferring her. He offered to enroll her in a Jenny Craig program and take her to the hospital to be weighed once a week since she couldn't stand on the bathroom scale. He also volunteered to cook low-fat dinners for them. Polly would enthusiastically agree, but within a few weeks Chuck would discover empty Oreo wrappers in the trash and demand an explanation. Polly denied all knowledge of how they got there. The ensuing arguments escalated into shouting matches that left them feeling humiliated and defeated, and their children bewildered and scared. Time and again, Chuck proposed new ideas for weight control, and Polly was always initially willing, but then began to cheat. Despite counseling sessions over the years, the conflict surfaced again and again. Chuck felt he made few demands on Polly, and couldn't understand why she was unable to do this one thing for him and their marriage—and for herself. He saw it as a rejection of him. They fought about Polly's eating up until she went to a nursing home. After she moved out, Chuck needed a year of counseling to resolve his anger at her, but in the clearer light of hindsight, he realized that food was Polly's therapy, and that for her, it was an irreplaceable pleasure. "That's where she got joy from," he says. "She didn't get it anywhere else."

Illnesses that cause mental changes present different but potentially even more dangerous challenges because they are less obvious and harder to assess. We have no idea how much to hold our spouses responsible for. Is their odd thinking deliberate, or the result of organic changes in their brains? How much of it can they help, and how much can they change? The answers are like feathers in the wind. Medical science can't help us here. Even sophisticated tests such as CAT and PET scans can't pinpoint whether the brain's emotion centers have been damaged.

Carly and Mike have a more recent bone of contention. With fifty-five-year-old Mike's breathing getting increasingly labored, Carly feels he won't live much longer. He has a life insurance policy based on the amount of his salary, but lately he has told the company bookkeeper to reduce it by half and pay Carly that amount so she can contribute to an IRA. "By the time I'm sixty-five, you'll have a nice IRA and all kinds of interest," he told her. Carly was flabbergasted. "Mike, even if you get a lung transplant, we're only talking about another three to five years," she said. Mike was outraged. "He started really screaming at me, and then he started gasping," she says. She walked away before the situation got serious. On this issue, unlike the automatic chair, Carly knows she can't win. She has gone to a counselor, who has taught her that she can change only her own behavior. She believes the lack of oxygen to Mike's brain has affected his judgment. "I'm powerless over his behavior, and I see his behavior as caused by his disease," she says. "He's just not himself. I have to let it go."

Sometimes denial looks a lot like hope, and a well spouse, out of love, sacrifices to allow it to continue. Margy Kleinerman's husband, Joe, was a professor of Spanish at a local college, but he spoke four other languages so fluently that he was also the foreign student advisor. At first, doctors couldn't account for Joe's shuffling gait and memory problems. They thought it might be hydrocephalus from a brain cyst he had as a child, but when it didn't progress in any predictable way, and after they had ruled out everything else, they diagnosed it as Alzheimer's. The disease had crept up on Joe slowly, over the course of ten years, mostly in the form of forgetfulness. "I told you about the wedding Saturday!" Margy would complain, while Joe would insist this was the first he'd heard of it. Or he'd claim that it was Margy's fault—if she weren't so gabby, he'd remember more of what she said, a claim Margy couldn't entirely refute. Only rarely would he admit, with a shake of his head, "Maybe I am getting forgetful." Joe's denial was so strong Margy couldn't bring herself to try to break through it. As long as Joe thought he had hydrocephalus, he consoled himself that he would recover. But Alzheimer's was so hopeless that Margy couldn't tell him about the changed diagnosis. Joe's denial became hers, until the night he almost killed them both.

Margy had never learned to drive and depended on Joe to take her everywhere. He sometimes forgot where a place was located, which concerned her, but he still seemed perfectly capable of driving safely. She ignored her friends' broad hints that Joe wasn't safe behind the wheel anymore. *He's been driving for so many years*, she told herself, *his driving is automatic by now. Besides, if I'm here, directing him, what could happen?*

The question was answered one night as they were driving to meet friends for dinner. Joe, formerly a man who risked getting a ticket for driving too slowly, turned into a speed demon, racing through a thirty-mile zone at sixty miles an hour. Margy was terrified. Joe didn't even seem to see the truck in the next lane, and missed hitting it by only a few inches. It got worse. He flew through a red light and nearly hit a car coming from the other direction. Margy, clinging to the dashboard, began to pray. "I think I'm losing control of the car . . . ," Joe faltered, and Margy realized he was pressing on the accelerator instead of the brake. "I said a prayer to a God I'm not even sure exists," she remembers. "I promised that if we got home safely, he'd never drive again." The next day, she had her daughter come over and take the car to her house. They told Joe it needed to be repaired.

The experience was a wake-up call for Margy, who realized she had been putting her life in danger by denying Joe's mental deterioration. When she heard of a friend of a friend who needed a place to live, Margy offered her room and board in exchange for chauffeuring and, until he went to a nursing home, helping her take care of Joe. She never could bring herself to tell Joe why the woman had moved in with them, though. "She just needs a place to live," she said. And she never told him he had Alzheimer's.

Keeping his illness a secret meant lonely isolation for her, because she could always talk to Joe about everything, but she believes it was the right thing for him. Talking to her three adult children, who understood and supported her, helped lessen the anguish of her decision.

Debbie Lang's situation was even more terrifying. Her husband, Dan, was only twenty-five, and she twenty-three, when he began having hand tremors. Two years later, he was told he had Parkinson's, but doctors were optimistic that since he was so young it would progress slowly and he could manage well with drugs.

From the outset, Dan denied. His mood swings and angry outbursts weren't his fault, he told Debbie. If the doctors could only get his medication adjusted, he'd be fine. Rather than provoke him, Debbie learned to tiptoe around, trying to keep their three little girls quiet so he wouldn't turn his wrath on them. The doctors told her that Parkinson's tended to emphasize a person's dominant emotions, and although Dan could be angry and domineering, she wasn't prepared for the way the illness exaggerated those tendencies. He went on spending sprees, draining the checking account so that there was no money for household expenses or clothes for the girls. He had the latest electronic gadgets and computers, but Debbie and the kids went without. He was never physically violent, but he was emotionally abusive, and intimidation made her give in to him rather than confront him. *Besides, he's sick*, she'd think. *He needs a little pampering.* She even made excuses for his behavior to his parents.

Over the next twelve years, he became angrier and more unpredictable, and life with him became a prolonged hell of shouting, violence, and constant vigilance. Telling Debbie "the doctors are stupid!" Dan increased his dopamine, which wreaked havoc with his mental state. She tried to hide the pills, even stashed them at her mother's house. He ferreted them out of closet shelves and the farthest reaches of dresser drawers, and charmed Debbie's mother into believing that Debbie had sent him over to get them. Too much dopamine made him paranoid, and he would wake Debbie out of an uneasy sleep. "There's someone outside the window staring at us," he'd say. "Go outside and check." When she tried to tell him no one was there, he called her a liar. Nighttimes were the worst. One night she and the girls were sound asleep when every light in the house went on. Dan jerked them out of their beds, screaming that they were trying to kill him. He ranted for hours, until, around 6:00 A.M., when she knew her parents would be up, Debbie grabbed the girls and ran to the car. After he began to make suicide threats, she packed up his gun collection and took it to her parents' house.

She still loved him, and tried to hang on, but her life became a bizarre carnival ride, with reassuring lulls alternating with cliff-hanging lurches toward disaster. During his calm times, she could almost convince herself that his medication was finally working properly and she could keep him home. He became the old Dan, the loving husband and father. Over time his behavior moved from frightening to downright dangerous. Dan, who had an electronics background, often slept during the day and conducted experiments in a back bedroom at night. Sometimes she awoke to the smell of propane filling the house, or he'd leave a hot iron on. She cried herself to sleep some nights, not knowing if they'd be alive in the morning.

Finally at her wits' end, she sent him to visit his parents in California. She was desperate for some peace, and thought Dan could be trusted with them. She and the girls were his targets; other family members didn't provoke him as they seemed to. With Dan out of the house, Debbie came to her senses. *This is how it should be*, she realized. *Not the war zone we've been living in.* Dan had been away less than two weeks when his parents called, asking her to come and get him. Dan had been terrorizing them too. Debbie arranged to have him admitted to Warm Springs, Montana's state mental hospital. He spent a year there. Only a week after he had been released to a local nursing home, he had put his fist through a window, thrown a wheelchair through another window, and kicked out a set of glass doors. He was transferred to the psychiatric ward of the local hospital.

She knew how manipulative he could be—it was one of the reasons she had been in denial for so long—but she was stunned when his psychiatrist called, telling her to come pick him up. "All he wants to do is come home to his family," the doctor explained. In disbelief, Debbie refused. The doctor became irate, telling her she was the one, not Dan, who needed psychiatric help. He insisted that once Dan was home he would be content and no longer disruptive. Debbie, horrified at the thought of Dan in their home again, began to recite the mayhem Dan had put them through in the past year. The doctor wasn't impressed. "You'll just have to deal with it, then," he told her.

Debbie didn't give in, but the words echoed. *Why can't I deal with it?* she wondered. *He's my husband. What's wrong with me?* She had finally gotten up the gumption to say "enough," and now one of Dan's doctors had joined him in his denial.

After several local nursing homes declined to take Dan, Debbie found one in another town. Even now, two years later, when they talk on the phone and he sounds normal, she thinks about bringing him home. Then she remembers. "Every time we've tried it, he's just blown it right out of the water," she says softly.

Debbie was a victim of "gaslighting" by Dan's psychiatrist. It's a well-known phenomenon among well spouses, the term taken from the movie *Gaslight*, in which Charles Boyer tries to convince Ingrid Bergman she's losing her mind. We find ourselves doubting our own sanity because our spouses present a deceptively normal picture to the rest of the world. They may manage to convince friends, family, or professionals that everything is fine, much to the dismay of the well spouse. One wife whose husband is on dialysis said, "People will ask him how he's doing and he'll say, 'Terrific!' and I want to put my hand up and say, 'Wait a minute . . .'"

Debbie Lang's case was egregious, but sooner or later, every well spouse will encounter a clueless mental health counselor, with no inkling of what it's like to live with someone with a chronic illness. As "helpers," counselors have a natural bias toward the sick person, and will put that person's needs first. They may cause our anxiety and depression to worsen because, due to their lack of experience, they believe we're exaggerating or overreacting. We then come away with the same set of problems as before, but now we also doubt our own responses to them. We may believe there's something wrong with us, instead of laying the blame squarely with our hopeless situations. Counselors can play critical roles in helping us through this ordeal—most well spouses say they couldn't survive without at least one—but we need to assess them carefully before trusting them with something as precious as our mental health. It won't be possible to find enough counselors who have firsthand experience themselves, though that would be ideal. The next-best solution is to make sure your counselor has the insight to make your point of view primary.

Family members' denial presents us with problems, too. In Chapter 4, we'll see how her children's denial drove a woman into the arms of another man. For their own peace of mind, family members need to believe a loved one is coping adequately, and sometimes our partners are surprisingly good at pulling themselves together enough to convince outsiders that they're functioning better than they actually are. A physician who treats Alzheimer's patients says he sees this situation all the time. The full-time caregivers are called hysterical and accused of overreacting when they talk about their fears. My husband's Uncle Charles, the one who had given us the down payment for our house, always told Don and me—and anyone else who would listen—how well Don was looking, up until a few weeks before he died. It became a sort of family joke that the better Charles said Don looked, the more we had cause to worry. I know now that Charles was indulging in a kind of magical thinking, as if pronouncing Don healthy would bring about the miracle he so desperately wished for his favorite nephew.

Indeed, denial in its milder forms can be a good thing. One of the subtle ways Don denied his illness was by using "we." "We're going to have to paint the house this summer," he might say, even though we both knew it was I, or the workers I hired, who would paint the house, not he. I didn't mind his use of the pronoun; I was touched that he still wanted to be involved in making decisions, even if he couldn't help carry them out. The little lie his "we" represented was a comforting form of denial, and one I conspired in. The difficulty for the well spouse is keeping the denial in balance, so that helpful denial is nurtured but destructive denial is challenged. Diane Maxwell says of Jim, "He has MS, and MS has him, and he fights a wheelchair because he doesn't want to give in, but he has given in to the mental demon of MS in so many ways. I don't want him to be in a state of denial, but I do want him to be in a state of reality."

While some people, on being told they have a chronic illness, go to bed and never get up, some are equally determined never to give in to it. Don was like that. He didn't deny that he had MS, but he denied adamantly, fanatically, that it was going to limit him. He loved his job as a property and casualty insurance underwriter and he was good at it. He liked trading banter on the telephone with agents around the state who sold his company's policies, and he enjoyed the interplay of personalities he worked with. His sense of humor made him well-liked. As the years of MS took their toll, and his fatigue got worse and worse, I wondered how he could possibly still be productive at work. He still worked an eight-hour day, even though I had suggested working part-time. "They'll have to tell me it's time," he told me firmly. "I'm not quitting." After much hesitation, I arranged a meeting with Ross, his immediate supervisor, at his home. I felt I had to know how Don was performing so that I could make plans, however tentative, for the future. Ross told me that Don was still pulling his weight, and I came away reassured, but I felt like a sneak and a traitor. What had this illness reduced us to, when I couldn't trust my own husband's perceptions on such a vital subject?

Don was able to continue to work for ten years after his diagnosis, and seldom missed a day because of illness. When the inevitable day came that the branch manager called him in and reluctantly told him he had to retire, Don was shocked. He was in such complete denial, he thought he was in line for a promotion. That night, I drove him home as usual in our handicapped-equipped van, and as I pulled into the driveway, he broke into tears as he told me what had happened. He was so shattered, I couldn't help crying too. He had loved his work. Now he was forty-two years old and unable to work anymore. Of all the cruelties this illness had subjected him to, this was one of the cruelest. I found out later that his coworkers sometimes had to lift his head from his desk and hold it upright. Sometimes he needed help getting out of the bathroom stall, and occasionally he had bowel and urine accidents at work. His speech on the telephone was hard to understand. Yet he believed he was a fully productive employee.

Often, our partners are fighting the demons of their illness so intensely that they develop tunnel vision. They simply don't see us anymore, or the fact that we've arranged the household to revolve around their needs. They deny that we have needs, or that our children do. When I began to broach the subject of a nursing home with Don, he was outraged. "All the way through this, you've only thought of yourself!" he shouted. In a calmer moment, I reminded him that every decision I made, and had made, since he got MS was based on what was best for him. When I pointed out that I drove him to work and picked him up, and worked a part-time job at home, so that I could be available to him, he looked abashed.

Diane Maxwell says that as Jim has gotten sicker, he often exhibits an attitude of "I am the only person in this room that matters. Meet my needs. I'm sick." Diane confesses that she can't tell whether that's the disease talking or Jim's self-centeredness. She was thrown into a tailspin last year when he announced, "I know the only reason you stay is for my disability pension." "My God," she replied, trying to keep her voice level, "after all the sacrifices I've made, that's what you think?" She fled to her church, empty that Easter Sunday afternoon, and cried for hours.

After many years of watching our partners get sicker, we come to realize there's only one way the journey will end. In the beginning, with an illness that can take an unpredictable course, we're optimistic. We cling to the hopeful reassurances of professionals, or the information produced by the disease associations, which sometimes glosses over the later stages of the illness and the grimmer statistics. If it's MS, we believe the literature put out by the MS Society, that MS doesn't shorten one's life, and that's what we tell our children. To be fair, these organizations have a difficult task addressing all the levels the illness can take. But their message can seem cruelly overoptimistic if your spouse happens to have a severe case. One woman whose husband has had MS for eighteen years says, "Our oldest daughter said to me once, 'Mom, you told us Dad wouldn't die of this disease.'" She explained to her daughter that that's what she and her husband had been told. She adds, "Those of us who are walking this road, though, you realize you do die of it, of the weakness or the pneumonia. You do die of MS. It's hairsplitting. The MS Society is in denial."

"You always think you have time," says Joan Fanti, whose husband, John, was quadriplegic for seven years after falling from a piece of equipment at work. John and his brother owned a sand and gravel company, and when one of the sifters broke, the two men climbed up on it and tried to fix it themselves. John only fell twelve feet, and he fell on sand, but neither of those things lessened the severity of his injury. At the trauma unit, doctors told Joan that John's neck was broken. They said that his spinal cord was still traumatized, but after the swelling receded, and with therapy, it was still possible he could regain movement in his body over the next two years. Joan clung to that hope, although John never improved. John had always been physically active and very fit, and although she saw his damaged body every day, she couldn't accept the image of him in a wheelchair, unable to feed himself. The Fantis told themselves that just because John was a quad didn't mean that he couldn't have a long life span. "John would say, 'In twenty years . . .'" says Joan, and she felt half-convinced herself, even though he was in constant pain and regularly being shuttled into and out of the hospital because of infections. Even the night he died, Joan assumed this hospital stay would be temporary like the others, and that John was not in danger of his life. After all, he had been joking with paramedics only ten minutes before he lapsed into a coma. Doctors had to warn Joan several times not to put John on a respirator. "They told me he wouldn't come off it," says Joan, who finally realized they were telling her this was the end.

Joan doesn't feel she missed anything by not being able to talk to John about his death ("He didn't believe in God anyway," she says), but talking honestly about death can allow us to lessen the inevitable guilt that follows a death. Pat Oswald says that before her husband, Fran, died of complications of Guillain-Barré, they "worked through everything." Fran even planned what food he wanted served at his funeral lunch.

Doctors, even though they're only guessing when they estimate how much time someone has left to live, can help our partners face their own mortality. Our family was fortunate that Dr. Shepard was willing to be liberal in interpreting the word "terminal." He reasoned that since Don could choke to death at any time, we were entitled to hospice services. Having hospice involved in our lives forced us to deal with the fact that Don's death could be imminent, and having a referral from a physician eliminated any possibility that we could tiptoe around the "elephant in the living room" any longer. With hospice counseling, the children and I were able to tell Don what he had meant in our lives, and how much we would miss him, and while this was an extremely painful time for us, it was enormously healing, too. (I'll talk about that time in more detail in Chapter 10.)

Families dealing with chronic illness must make the best of a medical profession that is geared toward short-term emergency care. Some organization analogous to hospice, with social workers, chaplains, and counselors, ought to exist now to assist our families—precisely because the sick spouse is not at death's door and the future looks so uncertain. Uncertainty is the most difficult aspect of living with chronic illness. The medical community must become more aware of the pressing emotional needs of families like ours, especially the need to communicate effectively with each other, and organizations must be designed to help us, even if the sick one is not yet *in extremis*. Eventually, perhaps, a team consisting of a social worker, psychologist, and medical professionals will be assembled when a diagnosis is given. For now, we have to take the initiative and assemble teams of our own.

Reach out to anyone you think might be helpful in assisting you or suggesting others who can. Our aging population is slowly growing into an awareness of the importance of counseling, consoling, and advising those with long-term illness and the families who love them.

Well spouses are in a tricky position when it comes to a partner's denial. Research shows that patients with higher levels of denial tend to cope better with chronic illness, so trying to tear down your spouse's denial system may not serve either of you in the long run. However, when denial becomes destructive, and it can become destructive when the well spouse can't talk about his or her needs, you may have to try to break through. Even if your partner hasn't reached the stage doctors refer to as "the dwindles," you're not facing reality if you don't acknowledge that death is an ever-present possibility. Someone whose coordination is off can fall; someone with respiratory distress or asthma can die of an attack; diabetics can slip into a coma; someone whose swallowing is compromised can choke to death. The rule to remember here is "Expect the best and plan for the worst." If you can't talk to your spouse directly, try to enlist the help of a physician who can frame the information in terms of "this may not happen to you, but here's what happens to most people with your condition." A realistic awareness of death is life-enhancing. Being able to talk to each other can bring a closeness that greatly diminishes the pain of loss.

# 3. Communication: A Gift in the Hand

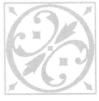Eugenia Staerker tells of an incident that characterizes the level of communication she has with her husband. Ray, age sixty-five, has had diabetes for fifty years, but in the past twenty-five years has had increasing complications, including a loss of vision. In 1980, he had his first laser treatment to cauterize blood vessels behind his eyes in order to prevent the tiny ruptures that cause blindness. Eugenia explains, "The first laser procedure, he didn't know what it was going to be like. It was awful, absolutely awful, very painful." He dreaded having another one, but the time came. "Of course, he knew from the first one what it would be like. And we're sitting there, in the doctor's office, and he says, 'I can't do this. I can't go through with it.'" On the spot, Eugenia made a decision. She got up and walked to the coat rack. Looking at her watch, she said, "OK then, let's go." Raymond looked at her in surprise. "He asked, 'Do you mean it?' and I said, 'Yes, but you'd better hurry and get your coat.'" He blinked. "What's the rush?" She replied, "The place

where you sign up for seeing eye dogs closes in about fifteen minutes." Ray's face changed. "You have such a subtle way about you, Eugenia," he grumbled softly. Then he laughed. "I guess I'll do it," he said. "I guess you want to see," she replied.

Eugenia says they have always been good communicators, which is why their thirty-two-year-old marriage is still mutually rewarding, in spite of Ray's increasing health problems. From the start, talk was something the Staerkers couldn't get enough of. "When we were dating, he said he didn't want to double date," she says, "because when you're with another couple you're not going to talk as much to each other. And the more you talk, the more you get to know each other." She and Raymond know each other, she says, "better than anybody."

"No misfortune without a gift in its hand" goes the saying, and nowhere is this more true than in the area of communication. One of the opportunities of chronic illness is the chance to deepen intimacy. At first, with the onslaught of terror and denial and depression that diagnosis dumps on us, we can't think clearly enough to talk to anyone—maybe not even ourselves. But as reality sets in, we realize, *This has happened. Nothing will undo it.* Couples who are able to turn toward, instead of away from, each other can become solid allies, building a marriage that unites them against a common enemy, helping them form a bond so strong that not even death destroys it. Illness blows the future to smithereens, and being able to comfort each other through that profound loss, and forge a satisfying relationship in the teeth of other relentless losses, is the best defense—maybe the only defense—we have against a hopeless situation. Couples who can negotiate this step will find that they know each other on a level they could never have imagined, one that many healthy couples never discover.

Unlike the Staerkers' enviable facility, Don's and my level of communication wasn't that good when we got married. He was fired from his job a few months after our wedding, and for weeks he withdrew into himself, a pattern I had seen when we were dating, when he thought he might be drafted and sent to Vietnam. Like many men, he couldn't, or wouldn't, talk about anything that really mattered. I felt confused and miserable, as well as useless in my new role as wife. Eventually he found another job and his spirits lifted. I also found out I was pregnant, and he was delighted.

Fast forward six years. When he began having trouble with walking and balance, and the possibility of MS darkened our lives, he reverted to his customary pattern of silence. I was pouring my heart out to counselors and psychiatrists, and taking tranquilizers, but I couldn't share my fears with the person who mattered most, my husband. We had quarreled several times about my frustration at his refusal to talk. One morning I heard the shower shut off, followed by, "Chrissie!" He was standing in the tub, dripping wet, immobilized by the fact that the edge of it had become too tall. "I'm scared," he said tearfully. "I'm afraid I'll fall getting out of here." "Stay there," I commanded unnecessarily. I got a kitchen chair and set it beside the tub, and he sat on it and lifted his feet over.

I look back on that moment as a turning point in our marriage. He literally stood naked before me. *This is what it's like for me*, he said wordlessly. *What are you going to do about it?* Somehow he trusted me not to laugh at him, or belittle him, or ignore him, or blame him because I expected him to be strong. For whatever reason, he had decided to share his illness with me. His MS had started to become ours instead of his. Without conscious planning, we had taken the first tentative steps toward real intimacy.

As the well one, I could have been the one who stopped talking. *He has so much on his mind*, I thought. *I won't tell him that I think about running away, that I'm afraid I'm too much of a coward to stay and watch this tragedy unfold.* But, more from a sense of self-preservation than any high-minded notion of what was good for my marriage, I couldn't keep quiet. I needed him. He was my best friend, the one I could show my worst self to, but who would, I had to believe, still love me, warts and all.

And MS certainly was revealing my warts. "You don't find out about yourself when things are going well," a friend tried to encourage me. "You only find out what you're made of when things go wrong." But the things I was finding out were the last things I wanted to know. Worrying about money, when my husband's medical care should be the most important consideration. Not wanting to come home in the evenings. Fantasizing about starting over somewhere else with a healthy man. Was this the "real" me? Didn't I have more character than that? I confessed these fears and feelings to Don, who, thank heavens, was understanding enough not to judge me either. We learned to say to each other, "I'm scared. I'm worried. I'm mad. I'm jealous," and not fear the other's reaction. Chronic illness forced us to trust each other.

Learning to bare your soul to another person means making yourself vulnerable, an act that can feel so frightening that even professional communicators find themselves stumbling into roadblocks they warn their patients against. Fran Willson, a psychologist, married her husband, Richard, also a psychologist, knowing he had polycystic kidney disease. She had been married the first time to a man who was "emotionally unavailable," but Richard was different. "I remember him saying, 'I don't know much about my future health. But I love you so much, even if I've only got ten years to live, I'd love to live them with you.'"

Her second marriage fulfilled all her dreams. "We can't imagine a better relationship in terms of caring and being there for each other, than we have," she says. Last year, Richard's condition worsened, and Fran was frightened. He slept a lot, awakened tired, and was losing weight. Good communication had been one of the greatest strengths in their marriage; still, Fran found herself unable to talk to him about her own fears, even though she was very troubled. Last summer, at a class she took on loss, the assignment was to make something in clay. "I thought what would come up was my first marriage, my parents' deaths, or other things," she says. "I was amazed that what my hands created, in all-white clay, was the form of Richard in a hospital bed. I couldn't stop the tears." Richard doesn't talk about his illness, she says, because "being courageous and dealing with this disorder, that's what keeps him going." She was afraid that sharing her own fears would break down that defense system, and she sees how well it works for him.

Although it took all her courage, she finally drove Richard to a beautiful spot along a river and began to talk. He told her he felt guilty because his illness was putting her through so much. "I said, 'That's helpful to hear, but all I wanted right now was for you to be able to hear my experience. I'm sorry you're feeling bad about that, but I think we need to hear from each other what's going on.' He really heard me out, and it was very helpful." Fran is surprised talking is so hard for them, two therapists. "We help a lot of people with medical problems, but it sure is different when it's your own."

We think of communicating in terms of words, but experts say up to 80 percent of it is nonverbal. Couples who have been together for many years may be very adept at reading body language and facial expressions, and have less need of conversation, because they know exactly how the other is feeling. Nor should we forget how important touch is in reassuring and comforting each other. I didn't realize, when Don went to the nursing home, how much he missed my touch until one day he admitted. "Some days I ache for you to just touch me." Under the circumstances, it seemed like little enough to do for him. Toward the end of his life, he'd say, "Put my arms around you," and I would do that. Some couples said they liked to lie beside each other in bed and just hold each other, even if they couldn't sleep in the same bed all night or have sex anymore. Our bodies have a language too, and it speaks volumes.

Listening without judging or criticizing is a useful marital skill, but it's essential when illness is involved. Establishing an atmosphere where both people feel free to be honest creates an oasis of safety within a terrifyingly uncertain situation. Just putting words to our bogeymen is like sticking a pin in them and watching them deflate—or at least shrink. Mark and Bonnie Johannes set aside time each week to talk. Initially a necessity, these sessions have become a blessing as well. "We share without argument, defensiveness, contradiction, or fear of accusation," says Mark. They've learned to avoid phrases like, "You make me angry when . . ." which puts the other person on the defensive. Mark says that their hard work—that's what it is—has deepened their understanding of each other, and their love, immeasurably.

Much miscommunication occurs because one person doesn't understand what the other person needs. By simply asking your partner for whatever it is, no matter how silly it seems, or how much you feel your husband or wife should know without your having to spell it out, you eliminate any possibility that he or she hasn't at least heard you. In one therapy group I heard about, well spouses and sick spouses role-played what they thought it was like to be the other, an eye-opener for both.

Understanding what the other person needs helps to avoid hurt feelings. Bonnie Johannes has learned not to feel shut out when Mark withdraws, because he sometimes needs solitude. His need to be alone might have caused problems for Bonnie, who refuels by being with people. Knowing these things about each other prevents either of them from feeling abandoned when they use their customary modes of comfort. Donna Keefe speaks of respecting each other's coping styles. "Pat can tell when I'm down. He just waits for me to get up again. When he's down, we talk." She says it's only been since his illness that he opens up and tells her what's the matter. Mark Johannes appreciates that Bonnie thanks him when he helps transfer her or gets her dressed. In return, he makes a point of complimenting her, and telling her he loves her, often. He respects her need to be self-sufficient, and doesn't automatically jump in to help unless she asks for it.

Eugenia Staerker agrees that kindness counts. "If my husband were abusive, I'd tell him right out, 'Don't ask me in that tone of voice.' Or I'd say, 'Do you mean, please get me this? Or, would I like to stop and get you that on the way home?'" Eugenia runs a well spouse support group, and tells about a woman, and there are many like her, who complained that her husband was never satisfied. "If she put the shade up, it's too much. I would tell that husband, 'Get a grip.'" "Yes, our spouses are sick," says Eugenia. "But I think they still need to be held to a standard of behavior."

The rules of courtesy apply to both spouses. When Don was in bed after his myelogram, I was waiting on him hand and foot—with little acknowledgment from him. "You know, it's your mother that's the nurse," I finally snapped. "But I'm not and I never wanted to be!" When I simmered down a little, I explained, "I'd like to be thanked more often for the extra work I'm doing," and Don made an extra effort. Years later, I was complaining about how much work he was. "I don't apologize," he said firmly. He was absolutely within his rights. He never asked to be so handicapped and had no control over his condition.

Open communication doesn't mean saying whatever comes

into your mind, especially when it involves complaining about the work load rather than problem-solving. We all know what one husband means when he says, "I bite my tongue a lot." But making an effort to talk to each other on topics other than illness can go a long way toward keeping love alive. With the daily drudgery of caregiving duties, we can lose sight of the unique human beings we married, turning him or her into a dirty rear, a hungry mouth, a pair of numb legs, while, in their eyes, we become animated fetching and carrying machines. By keeping the lines of communication open, partners can, and must, remind each other that they still have souls.

Holding each other to a certain standard of behavior is particularly important if the sick spouse starts to become abusive. Because we may empathize, to an unhealthy degree, with their suffering, we allow them to take out their anger on us. That's a mistake. As Mark Johannes says, "We're responsible only for our own feelings. I can't make her feel better, and she can't make me feel better." Many spouses fall into the trap of assuming responsibility for their partner's emotional state as well as physical well-being, a staggering load—and an unfair one, believes Shevy Healey, a clinical psychologist who counsels couples dealing with illness. "Well spouses often fall into two categories," she says. "They either walk on eggs around the partner for fear of offending them, or putting them into depression, or they're angry around them all the time. There seems to be no way they're not triggered by whatever the partner is doing. That's symbiosis of the worst kind." She says, "I would support a well spouse who says 'I'm not going to take your anger anymore.'"

While the limitations chronic illness imposes sometimes seem insurmountable, a marriage comprises two lives, not one. Each person is responsible for finding ways to live to the fullest, illness notwithstanding. Sick spouses aren't off the hook because they're sick. "The price of nice" will soon bankrupt a spouse who doesn't set limits on a partner's behavior. Eugenia Staerker says that when Ray insisted the garbage can be flush with the wall, a nicety that mattered not a whit to her, she told him it was up to him to put it there. "So now the can's flush with the wall," she says.

Nor is the sick partner always the nasty one. One husband with heart disease ordered his wife out of their house because he couldn't cope with her negativism any longer. He had enough to deal with, he said. Caregivers constantly need to assess their own limits in regard to their partners, what psychologists call "defining boundaries," and then make sure they understand where our compassion ends. Otherwise, we become enablers of a partner's chronically offensive behavior. What we permit, we promote.

Learning where our limits are is part of the psychological work of being a well spouse, and it can take years. Natalie, whose husband, Dennis, has had diabetes since his teens, says she was raised to be the perfect daughter. "I was the only girl of my generation on both sides of my family," she says. "We didn't yell or scream." She had to learn how to define her own needs, and her therapist taught her how to tell him about them. And, like most ill spouses, he needed lots of telling. One of the big pleasures in her week is her Sunday morning golf game with a friend. "Then we go to breakfast, and schmooze, and it's very relaxing. It's become a ritual," she says. At first, he objected. "Dennis would like me to be here more, but I'm very clear that this is something I need to do for me. There's been a lot of talking, and a lot of discussing. And a lot of yelling. I had to learn how to yell." Finally he realized she came back feeling better, and saw how those Sunday mornings restored her. But they still disagree about how she spends her time. "Sometimes he'll say, 'I don't want you to do such and such,' and I'll say, 'I'm aware of that, but I'm going to do it anyway.'" One of the rules of good communication is that Person A doesn't have to like what Person B is doing, but they are able to tell each other in ways that are not hurtful.

Natalie says Dennis's behavior "is better in many ways than it's been," because she's set clear boundaries. Along the way she also learned to control her anger. "I say, 'I understand that you're sick, and that is not good, but I'm not going to accept this behavior.' He'll start yelling and hollering, and I say, 'I'll be happy to listen to you, but not if you're yelling.' I have very definite limits."

Hilde got tough when her husband, Hank, injured in a car accident, came home from "rehabilitation." What happened, to Hilde's thinking, was that the facility threw up its hands and decided he was someone else's problem. Hank came home a savage, noncommunicative, incontinent man given to unpredictable rages during which he would try to claw her and bite her whenever she approached. With no money for a nursing home, Hilde knew she was the last stop, but if she was to care for him, she had to tame him. When Hank tried to attack her, she left the room. "I would slam the door really loud so that he could hear it," she says. "I said, 'If you calm down, I might come back.'" After a while, she could hear the penitence in his voice, and after a longer while, decipher his words: "Mommy, I be good." Then she'd go back in. Her refusal to be bullied paid off, although it took two years. "I had to learn I don't just slap the washcloth in his face," she says. "I had to tell him, I'm going to wash your face now. See, here's my hand, here's the washcloth, I'll put it in your face now and rub your face with it." Her experience shows that even someone with limited cognitive functioning can be persuaded to behave acceptably.

If your partner can't be civil, you may have to remove yourself from the fray. Barbara Beachman says that even from the nursing home, her husband, Chuck, still tries to run her life. "I have some bad times when he gets very controlling and very mad," she says. Last summer he became verbally abusive when she wouldn't account for her time down to the minute. "I had to put a call block on my phone for three months," she says. When their kids questioned her, she played one of Chuck's messages back for them. "Oh, God, Dad's off the wall," said one. The old Barbara would never have had the nerve; the new Barbara takes care of herself.

Of course, when an illness brings on memory and cognitive problems, communication is impaired, maybe impossible. For Margy Kleinerman, communication mixups with her husband, Joe, were the first sign of his Alzheimer's disease. He had always had a phenomenal memory, but suddenly he couldn't remember things she'd told him yesterday. Only when he forgot the route to the school where he'd been teaching for fourteen years did it dawn on her that something was seriously wrong.

Ironically, in one case, a wife didn't discover for years that her husband's verbal ability concealed subtle brain injuries. Rhoda's husband, John, who had a stroke and subsequently developed seizures, never lost his vocabulary. Rhoda says, "His ability to converse at a very high level masked a lot of cognitive deficits, because he could talk to you. It took me a long, long time to figure it out, that the affect was definitely off." Repeatedly, John made promises he never kept, and Rhoda decided to divorce him. Communicating isn't a panacea if your spouse only talks about changing but never follows through.

One woman whose husband has had MS for twenty years says, "He has a way of changing the subject in mid-sentence so I have to say, 'Whoa, whoa, whoa.' It's frustrating. I just say, 'Wait, let's start over.' The other day I said, 'Reggie, talking to you is so frustrating because I really want to have a serious discussion about this, and you keep losing the thread of the conversation and launching off on some other tangent. And he says, 'I know, I know.' I think he's aware of it, but can't help it. It's like a short circuit." The psychologist she goes to helped her understand that he really can't help it—and that has helped her. "You don't tell somebody to run up the street if they're hobbling along on a broken leg." Although, for her, making all the decisions is one of the most burdensome things about being a well spouse, she's decided she must. "But I hate feeling responsible for everything."

The heartache of losing our most precious confidant, a husband or wife, goes deep. Another wife, an eighteen-year veteran of the MS wars, says, "Our conversations are pretty superficial. Sometimes I'll get started on something that happened at work, and I'll just lose him. He'll say, 'I don't know what you're talking about.' I don't get angry. I just say, OK." She says sadly, "When you're married to someone for thirty-five years, you can just about start a sentence and know what the other's going to say. But more and more, I just can't get across to him." She has learned to look elsewhere for intellectual stimulation and emotional intimacy.

Some couples find that poking fun at life's ridiculous side can be the sharpest knife in the drawer when it comes to cutting problems down to size—not the easiest thing to do, but worth the effort. Humor creates distance between us and whatever is dragging us down, and some spouses find their sense of humor becomes honed by well spousedom because it's a sanity-saver. Making fun works especially well on hated but necessary equipment. Don told me that when he was a child, his mother read him stories about a family called *The Happy Hollisters*. So when he began using condom catheters manufactured by a company named Hollister, what else could we call the nasty little things but his "happy hollisters"? Bonnie Johannes recently started using a urinary overnight bag, which she refers to as her "new pull toy." Not to be outdone, Mark refers to it as her "boat anchor." Well spouse humor often arises because if we don't laugh, we'll cry. Mark Johannes says that once when Bonnie was making Chinese food, her knees buckled and she ended up on the floor, covered with sticky sauce. "I said, 'Oh, you look good in sweet and sour sauce.' It's still funny to us." Shared laughter says: We're on the same side, and no matter how bad things get, we're stronger than this mess we're in.

Pat and Fran Oswald took the gallows humor to Fran's bedside after he became quadriplegic with Guillain-Barré. In fact, even Fran's doctor told them how much he admired their ability to see humor in everything. What had happened to Fran was so sudden and so devastating, Pat says, "we used to say, 'Boy, we must have been some beauts in our past lives to be dealing with all this heavy stuff.'" Pat recalls, "I would say, 'Fran, this is a disease Hitler should have gotten. But why you? You never hurt anybody.'" Then she'd tease, "But you must have been bad in a past life," and they'd laugh. Linda Anderson says that Steve, who had MS when they got married, "had a wonderful sense of humor. It gets you through a lot. Some of the things that seemed most depressing, we'd make jokes about." She knew that she and Steve had to be careful of shocking people who overheard their jokes. "You can't say certain things around everyone."

Not only must we learn new ways of talking to our spouses; we must also learn new ways of talking to people in our communities. Spousal illness throws new roles at us faster than we can blink. Now we are the ones who must arrange bank loans, argue with insurance providers, question doctors, learn the inner workings of a car engine. Each of these roles means learning a new vocabulary.

Nothing has prepared us for becoming a spouse's advocate, but when they are too sick or too injured to speak for themselves, that job falls to us. Even though we cry in private, we have to present a brave face to the world. Is it any wonder that some days we're ready to check into the nearest asylum? Debbie Lang sometimes finds herself thinking, "Get the bed ready next to Dan's, I'm moving in." Especially for women, a partner's illness may be the first time we've had to stand up for ourselves, and the role feels strange and uncomfortable. But when we look around to see who else is going to do it, no one is there.

No one comes to well spousehood knowing how to do this job. We acquire these skills by doing them. Because Pam Cook was a certified nurse's assistant before her husband, Don, was seriously brain-injured in an explosion at the fertilizer plant where he worked, she trusted the doctors who treated him at the rehabilitation facility. But after finding him lying in his own feces, and sleeping most of the time because of the powerful narcotics he was on, she learned to speak up. Her sister helped her, too. "She'd say, 'This is Don they're talking about here. What do you think?'" After Pam demanded he be taken off the drugs, he came out of his coma, which surprised the doctors, but not Pam. Soon she had him off the tracheostomy tube, too. "Before, I was told what to do, when to do it, and how to say it. But Don had been so good to me, I thought, I've got to stand up for him."

Getting assertive has helped in her ongoing battle with the insurance company. Because her husband's injury was covered by worker's compensation, each expenditure she makes for him must be approved in advance. "They're the rudest people I've ever met in my life," she says. "They make up the rules as they go along." She's had to take them to court twice and is considering a third time. Since she's a CNA herself, she expects Don's nurses to be capable. "The most stress in my life comes from the nurse's aides," she says. "Some of them don't want to do certain things, some only come for the money, and some don't know what to do, so I have to teach them. I know what they learn, so they're not kidding me."

We've never been well spouses before, yet we believe we should know how to do it—perfectly, the first time. When we blame ourselves for failing, we're being unfair to ourselves. People in the helping professions, such as Fran Willson, know how paralyzing these expectations can be. Another woman, a social worker, told me, "I felt I was supposed to know how to do this because of my job. I didn't get nearly the help I needed because pride held me back." Seeking out resources can be a special hurdle for men, who may believe they are supposed to know what to do—especially if they're in charge at their jobs. Your local hospital can refer you to support groups, which can be excellent sources of information and shortcuts. They also serve as grapevines that can keep you informed of changes in laws and government red tape. Groups like these can also provide the encouragement you need to set limits on a spouse's behavior. Finding out what others will and won't tolerate from their own spouses helps you decide whether your partner is out of bounds or whether you're overreacting.

Communicating clearly comes from being able to see clearly, and we all know how difficult that can be when you're in the middle of the maelstrom. A good counselor can help you define your priorities as a well spouse. This person will probably be a professional, and may also be a current or former well spouse, someone whose opinion you respect, and, above all, a good listener. I was greatly helped by the fact that my most helpful counselors over the years were Catholic like me, although religion or spiritual orientation may not matter to you. Counselors may be clergy, hospice workers, social workers, psychologists, or psychiatrists. Talking to friends can bring release, but it can also be problematic. Natalie says that her therapist is more capable of helping her see both sides of an issue because her friends are, naturally, biased in her favor. Another woman mentioned that while her friends were willing to listen to her problems, they didn't share their own because "theirs seemed so trivial." Be aware that your friends may have this perception, even if they don't tell you about it. As in any other profession, therapists come in all degrees of competency, but a lot of degrees don't guarantee competency. A relationship like this should, above all, feel right. How does this person conduct his or her own life? Would you respect him if he weren't your therapist? Do you like him or her personally? If you're not satisfied, keep looking. I am convinced that some of the people who came into our lives during the course of Don's illness did nothing less than save our lives, while others were remarkably useless. Trust yourself if someone doesn't feel right for you. I once went to an appointment with a social worker who turned out to be a twenty-one-year-old man. I walked right out again and insisted on talking to someone nearer my age, and female. The young man may have had the wisdom of Solomon, but I doubt it. We give so much ourselves that sometimes we have to demand that someone give to us.

If you decide on couples counseling, keep in mind the therapist will have a natural tendency to favor your sick partner. I had an infuriating encounter with a counselor Don had gone to first. When I confided to her that I often thought about leaving, I expected her to listen and help me sort out my feelings. Mostly, I just wanted to rant for a while. But she had come to admire Don, and decided I was the flaky wife about to abandon her helpless patient. Beware of falling into traps like this one. As Mark

Johannes deadpans, "Our marriage counselor really helped us. He became a common enemy."

As bad as the bad counselors can be, the good ones are priceless. Both by inclination and training, I'm someone who puts great stock in the power of language. I learned, over the course of this experience, however, that sometimes words fail. They aren't adequate to encompass all the emotions involved, and they wear out. When you've had the same conversation with your spouse a hundred times about whether it's time for a nursing home, for example, you feel like you're trudging, yet again, over the same barren ground. One of the unusual ways a counselor helped Don and me, and our children, was by devising rituals that helped us through transitions. Because well spouses' lives are full of frustrating "ambiguous losses," difficult to define and consequently difficult to grieve, acknowledging them with rituals can help us past feeling stuck and unable to move on. When Don entered the nursing home, a counselor had all of us, including the children, exchange pink, rose-scented candles. We could burn our candles when we wanted to be reminded of each other's love. The ceremony said so much more than "Good-bye" and "We love you," although it said those things too. It marked the end of our lives under one roof and acknowledged that Don would be living elsewhere now. The value of ritual is that it takes the burden off words that have become tired and worn out, by involving our bodies and as many of our five senses as possible. Ritual says things words can't say.

A few years later, the same counselor helped Don and me exchange modified wedding vows, telling each other that our marriage was no longer the one we had entered into so many years ago, and helping us free each other "to live in our separate worlds." This ritual helped me pick up the pieces of my life when my husband could no longer be the loving sexual partner he had been. Good counselors can become the midwives who coach us through the intense pain that accompanies growth.

The personal counseling I got helped me keep my equilibrium and lessened the scarring from this experience. If ever a life situation called for many different kinds of helpers with many different kinds of vision, this is it. We see the barriers only too well. We need people around us who can help us see the possibilities.

# 4. Sex:
# The Plaster Saint
# Syndrome

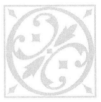 Sex is the glue that holds a marriage together. Discovering that no aspect of our lives, even the most intimate, is safe from illness is shattering. I remember staring at the ceiling after an unsuccessful try at lovemaking, and raging inwardly, *This part should be off-limits, dammit! Leave us something!* I was outraged and devastated.

Don had been tentatively diagnosed with MS when he began having problems with impotence for the first time in our marriage. He had no idea what might be causing it; although the myelogram had left him with lingering headaches, mostly he was feeling well.

I was terrified that the MS was already beginning to affect his sexual functioning, although it seemed awfully early for that. He was somewhat unsteady on his feet, but that was the only sign of the MS. There was no definitive way of finding out, either. Even the most sensitive medical test would not have been able to tell us whether the plaques of scar tissue that caused MS had wrapped themselves around the nerves responsible for an erection. No such medical test existed then, or now.

I thought it more likely that Don's problem was psychological—that he was worried about his future with me, his job, his health—even his life. I had just started teaching English part-time at a local college, and one night I had a Coke with one of my male students. I had never lied to Don, and didn't see any reason to now. I told him where I had been. When he blew up, I saw how afraid he was. He must have feared that he stood to lose not just his health, but his wife, his children, everything he believed was his.

Certainly that kind of fear could cause impotence. And although spending an hour after class in a well-lighted cafeteria with a student could hardly be described as wanton, some of my thoughts were not so pure. I was still young; my classes were filled with men of all ages. *Maybe I can erase this chapter of my life*, I thought, *take the kids and start over with one of the healthy bodies I see all around me.* Confiding these thoughts to Don was out of the question. He had enough to deal with. I wasn't about to add to his worries.

To compound the situation, he began to want sex more often. He needed to reassure himself that he was still OK; I needed to withdraw and consider the steep turn my life had taken. We argued. One night he put a fist through the living room wall.

Eventually the situation righted itself. I realized how much I loved him. I had escape fantasies, but I didn't want anyone else. As much as I wished it were a healthy body, it was still *his* body I wanted. Time allowed us to absorb the shock of the diagnosis, and we were able to talk about our fears. I reassured him that I wasn't going anywhere, but that sometimes I would need to retreat. The impotence went away, only to return sporadically toward the end of his life.

When so much energy must be directed at the discomforts, medications, treatments, and worries of a chronic illness, there isn't much left for whispering sweet nothings. A woman whose husband has kidney disease says, "I think the illness is the sick spouse's mistress. It's the first thing he thinks about when he wakes up—'How am I feeling today?' and the last thing he thinks about when he goes to bed—'How do I feel now?'" She continues, "If she is in a bad mood, his day is shot. She's very controlling. When we go out, it's not the two of us, but the three of us. She walks between us when we walk side by side, but more often, she walks beside him [i.e., his cane] and I trot along behind them."

If only talking about this vital part of our lives weren't so difficult. We are acutely aware that a significant portion of our partners' self-esteem resides in sexual performance and desirability. Because we're afraid of hurting them, we don't talk, and they imagine the worst. It's a vicious cycle: The intimate sharing that follows sex would allow a place and time to talk about fears and fantasies, but we need a certain amount of intimacy to have satisfactory sex in the first place. Just as it dawns on us how many problems are resolved in bed, the problem becomes the marriage bed.

Experimenting with new techniques, and talking about difficulties, may work well early in the illness when the problems are more likely to be psychological, but as an illness progresses, physical factors are more likely the cause of problems. Some illnesses, or the medications they require, may compromise or eliminate sexual functioning. Diabetes and MS are two that alter sensation, causing loss of orgasm for women and impotence for men. As an illness progresses, experimenting feels riskier because more is at stake. We don't want our partners to think we're criticizing, even though the old ways may not work anymore. Then too, the precious emotional equilibrium we have with our mates is fragile. If we try to have sex and fail, it may depress both of us further.

One of the biggest taboos is admitting we're turned off by the changes in a partner's body. Hollywood loves the myth that suffering is glamorous, and that people sicken and die beautifully. But then, you never see anyone emptying bedpans or cleaning up vomit on the big screen, either. Jim Russell says of his wife, Hannah, "I mean, I have to bathe her, put her on the commode, clean her up, she's basically quadriplegic, she can't do anything." He says, "She still expresses a desire for closeness. I know closeness doesn't mean having sex. But when you do this day in and day out, when you're woken up two or three times every night, it's like, now I'm going to make love to this woman? Give me a break." Caring for the body we used to find sexy changes our feelings for it. As one husband said poignantly, "I can't have sex with my wife because it feels like incest. She's my child."

A man whose wife has a spinal cord injury put it more starkly. "We were living in Milwaukee, and I don't know if you remember Jeffrey Dahmer, that case? He was a necrophiliac. Jolene and I were making love one time, and it was during all the publicity about Dahmer, and I felt like I was having sex with a dead person. I just stopped. She asked why, and I couldn't tell her. I said something like, it wasn't satisfying. I wasn't getting any pleasure out of it anymore."

Whether we are able to maintain a sex life may depend on other factors besides physical ability. Some partners don't want to experiment. One wife says that after her husband's strokes, "I didn't want to explore other ways of having sex. That was probably wrong of me, but I'm very squeamish."

I found that maintaining some flexibility about what "good

sex" meant brought rewards. Although I mourned the loss of the good old missionary position with my husband, I wasn't ready to call it quits, and neither was he. I was surprised to find that wheelchair sex, rather than feeling like a loss, expanded our sexual repertoire. After I realized there was no way to be graceful, I felt free to enjoy myself. After he became paralyzed, I would ask him to describe what he would be doing to me if he could. Sometimes I had to fight back tears, but these descriptions were arousing for both of us. I realized how powerful language is, and that, indeed, the brain is the most important sex organ.

Another reason I held on to physical intimacy for so long was that when Don and I were horizontal, I could forget about the illness that invaded the rest of our lives. No wheelchair diminished him by half. He was exactly my height. Lying down, face to face, looking into his eyes, talking as we always had, we were equals. I couldn't bear to let that go, and I didn't.

Illness can bring unwanted psychological changes as well as physical changes in the partner we loved. If, as sometimes happens, a husband or wife becomes selfish, abusive, and demanding, having to have sex with him or her feels like acceding to one more demand. Chronic illness leaves a caustic residue of anger, because, as Elisabeth Kubler-Ross writes, "The process of grief always includes some qualities of anger." The sick one may be furious he is sick; the well one may be frustrated at being turned into a full-time caregiver. Each blames the other, and nothing kills desire faster than anger. Add in the sheer exhaustion that comes from the duties of caregiving, and the result is not exactly a recipe for romance. Linda Anderson's husband, Steve, had MS when they married, and as she "made the transition from part-time caregiver to full-time caregiver," her interest in sex waned. She says, "Emotionally, sex was a difficult thing to give up. That was a connection, part of what made us a couple, that you can't describe. I was still in love with him, but there wasn't that desire anymore."

The sex-role changes necessitated by illness alter our ability to feel manly or womanly. One woman whose husband has kidney disease believes that illness has castrating effects on the couple, not just on the sick person. "He gets more feminine as he gets sicker, and she, the well spouse, has to take on more and more masculine qualities as she must do all those things the man would traditionally do." According to her, well wives "simply don't have the luxury of being feminine—no time, no opportunity, no acknowledgment. The sick husband actually becomes womanly—whining, delicate, neurotic, while the well wife takes on manly characteristics."

In chronic illness we grieve the loss, not just of sexual function, but of sexuality. We lose the opportunity, encouragement, luxury—the joy—of expressing the masculine or feminine part of ourselves. Sex, with its rich layers of memories and associations, is so much more than a physical act. It allows a sharing of our deepest selves that doesn't occur at any other time. Losing a sexual partner means losing the appreciation of our sexuality, from both them and ourselves. We lose the awareness of our desirability and attractiveness. We lose self-esteem.

It hurts, this loss that hauls along a trailerload of other losses. Norma Imber says that she and Robert "had a perfect sex life, very warm and tender and loving. It was very caring. It was perfect." Another woman says eloquently, "My feeling about the 'S' subject is like a newly armless man pondering his former career as a diamond cutter. Which gives you a very clear idea of where this happy couple is on that subject."

Sexual activity began to feel like one more chore for Roy Layton, who was caring for his wife, Donna, with MS. He remembers, "What it amounted to was that it had become another demand on me. She still would have been agreeable, but I reached a point where, between my anger and frustration and exhaustion, the very idea of putting out the effort involved in some sort of distorted representation of intimacy, I just found appalling. I just couldn't stand the thought. It was sort of a mockery of an intimate relationship."

Stopping the sex can be a painful turning point, because our partners have so few pleasures in their lives and we hesitate to take away something else. Even after her husband, who has diabetes, became impotent, Georgina continued with oral sex, an acceptable substitute for both of them. "Then it got to the point where it wasn't enjoyable," she says. "It was for him, but not for me. I finally told him I didn't want to keep doing it. I tried to explain to him that it was impossible for me to be attracted to his body on a sexual level because I was taking care of every aspect of his body. I had to work up the courage to tell him, but I felt I was doing enough for him, and I just couldn't give sexually anymore." Predictably, her husband was dejected. "I don't want to use the word devastated," she says, "but he was unhappy. I tried to explain that I didn't find him unappealing, but it still hurt his self-esteem." At the time, she felt guilty. "I felt he was being cheated more than I, because I had other aspects of my life. Now I realize we were both cheated."

John Rolland, M.D., whose first wife died of cancer at age thirty, is the author of *Families, Illness, and Disability*. He states, "For someone who expresses intimate feelings mostly through sexuality, a partner's illness can create a serious crisis. This is more common among men than women." Mary Lambert, a licensed psychotherapist in New York City, was a well spouse herself for seven years after her husband suffered a serious stroke. She says that men rarely want to give up sex. "It's mostly the women who want to withdraw," she says. This holds true whether the woman is the well spouse or the sick one. "For men, this is like Custer's Last Stand." She smiles. "I mean to make a pun. It's usually women who say to their husbands, let's forget it."

One wife says that her husband, even from a nursing home, "doesn't ever stop thinking about sex. Finally one day I said to him, 'Let me ask you a question. Do you really think you could? Tell me the truth.' And he said 'No.' And I said, 'Then let's not talk about it anymore, because it really makes me feel very sad.'" Like many husbands, hers is "stable but unable."

If men associate touching only with sex, they may stop touching completely, as Diane Maxwell found. "I miss the closeness. It isn't the orgasms, it's the cuddling. Jim used to do it, but since he can't perform, he doesn't do it anymore. Maybe it reminds him."

So we struggle to keep this vital part of our marriages going, and don't surrender it without great regret. But in spite of our best efforts, the day comes when we realize we have become celibate. What to do about sexual deprivation is a big question. Some believe the only answer is abstinence: "If you read the Bible, you'd know," wrote one correspondent to the newsletter *Mainstay*. For some, becoming celibate is a less painful decision than for others. For these couples, companionship was always more important than sex. For others, the loss is huge. Men, with their stronger sex drives, may be more inclined to find new sexual partners than women—and because of their jobs, may have more opportunities to do so. Length of marriage, as well as age, is a factor too. Older people who enjoyed an active sex life for years often accept celibacy with good grace, or at least better grace than younger ones who thought marriage came with a guarantee of regular sex. A man whose wife developed Parkinson's symptoms shortly after they were married says, "It was probably the loneliest thing in the whole wide world. You put the kids to bed, you put her to bed, and there's nothing left. You've done your thing for the day."

Illness cheats us out of so many things we expected to share with our mates that we may feel entitled to seek satisfaction elsewhere. But we may also find ourselves agonizingly divided about whether to act on that belief. A woman who attended a weekend caregivers' gathering says, "I was ambivalent about the couples that formed over the weekend. My first reaction was fear. I thought, 'Oh dear, I don't want to do that. I want to keep my marriage vows.' But I forced myself to look at it, and had real mixed emotions. I thought, 'How do you spend the weekend with this person, then go back to your chronically ill spouse?' Somehow, in my mind, that would make it harder." Others find the idea of an affair laughable—where would they find the time? When you're working a job, raising kids, and taking care of a sick husband or wife for the few hours left in the day, there's hardly time for a trip to the bathroom, much less the time and energy another relationship would require.

One woman, whose husband has had diabetes for twenty-two years, says, "I'm not interested in other men. It's not a no-no, it's just a no-interest. I just don't want to get involved in an emotional relationship that's going to drain me." Understandably, many well spouses feel too overextended emotionally to take on something as potentially volatile as an affair.

But the alternative, celibacy, feels like swimming upstream against a sexy culture. We already feel isolated; becoming celibate isolates us even more. We look out on a world full of healthy couples who can have sex anytime they want, or so it seems. Our culture bombards us with the notion that sex is a necessity, rather than one pleasure among many. We can easily become convinced that we're watching the best years of our sexual lives dribble away. As one man wrote to *Mainstay*, "I sometimes feel like that starving Charlie Chaplin character who is looking through the restaurant window, watching overweight diners stuff themselves."

For some with strict religious convictions, the message is clear: They had the bad luck to choose a partner who became ill, so now they must live with the consequences. We may believe that our friends and neighbors expect us to surrender our sexuality too, in order to conform to society's model of "good" husbands and wives. I remember as a teenager the condemnation heaped on a male family member who sought female companionship after his wife became paralyzed. I shared their disapproval—until I found myself in his situation many years later. Then I was angry. *What right,* I thought, *had any of us to judge him?*

Sexuality is part of our identities as men and women, so we can't lose it, even if we lose the opportunity to express it. But a woman who describes her husband as a "kidney cripple" speaks of a psychological numbness that comes from repressing that part of her personality for so long. "There has never been an affair, nor has there ever been a temptation. I just can't imagine that anyone would ever think of me in such a way. Of course, if someone did, I probably wouldn't even recognize the signs."

Many well spouses learn to, in Freud's terminology, "sublimate." They spend more time with children or grandchildren, travel, or take up hobbies. When our partners can't have sex anymore, it's often the hugging, touching, cuddling, and sitting on a warm lap that we miss, more than the sex act itself. We may have to tell our partners that those things are still important, even if sexual intercourse is impossible. Activities that involve tactile stimulation, such as pottery, quilting, and gardening, can be especially satisfying distractions. Mental hospitals have long understood the calming effects of hand crafts like basket-weaving and painting. For several years after Don went to the nursing home, I had regular massages, which reminded me that I was still sensual, in addition to making me feel pampered. For many, masturbation can be a satisfactory alternative, and doesn't entail the risks of disease, commitment, or scandal. Turning to drinking or eating, while temporarily soothing, only creates other problems. A woman whose husband developed Parkinson's at a young age says, "Some people drink and some people smoke, but I took to eating and became a heavyweight." She wonders if that was deliberate. "I think I've kept this appearance because if I looked good, somebody might be interested, and that would be wrong. 'Cause I'm still Christian, and when you're married, you're married for life."

Still, we wonder, what if someone came along? Time and again, well spouses say that sex is important, but the question of what comes next leaves us in a haze of confusion and doubt. Would it hurt our spouses if we had an affair? Would it hurt us? What about our children?

John Rolland writes that the question of extramarital relationships stumps clinicians, too, "because standards applied to physically healthy couples may not fit the excruciating long-term strains of couples facing illness and disability." Rolland himself does not advocate affairs. "I have seen many instances in which an affair was destructive and hastened the end of a relationship. I have also seen a number of instances . . . in which an affair allowed a well partner to sustain his or her commitment to caring for a spouse."

Of all the questions well spouses must answer for themselves, the question of whether to have an affair is the most intensely personal. Each of us has a unique set of values and religious beliefs, and we move in our own orbits of social, family, and work relationships, so we must be the sole decision-makers here. We alone must live with the consequences.

Nor is the question settled once and for all. Meeting someone who is interested in us sexually may change our minds, as we'll see later in this chapter. And just the wearing down of life with a chronic illness can change our point of view over time. A woman whose husband is seriously disabled with diabetes says, "I wouldn't have considered an affair initially, but I've changed. I think the initial feeling, that that would be a terrible thing to do, I'm a terrible person, was wrong. It wouldn't make me a terrible person, it just means I'm missing a piece of my life. I wouldn't take any less good care of my husband than I do now."

She has been able to put the sexual part of herself in perspective, to see it as a legitimate human need. But not all of us can be so practical. Not wanting to violate one's own values is a very big hurdle; but even if we can justify a liaison to ourselves, we turn and confront the rest of the world—family, neighbors, and friends. What will they make of our friendships with the opposite sex? Because of our spouses, we may feel fairly visible in our communities, especially if we live in small towns. If we have an affair, we think, everyone will know—and we'll fall from our pedestals with a crash. In sexual matters especially, well spouses are victims of the "plaster saint syndrome," because everyone wants to idealize us for our devotion to our sick partners. According to the prevailing thinking, nothing, certainly not our own sexual needs, should interfere with our higher purpose of caregiving. Because the rest of the world sympathizes with our spouses, it may judge us harshly for having an affair. Fidelity, on the other hand, earns us universal admiration, and we may hesitate to surrender one of the few perks in our lives. "Everyone thinks of me as a saint," wrote one *Mainstay* correspondent. "What will they think if I have an affair?"

"I'd like to meet someone after Robert dies," says Norma Imber. "But I don't feel comfortable dating now, because the other ladies I know would kill me. They'd say, 'You're married. You have a husband.' They'd say that."

Ironically, her family's stubborn refusal to see that her marriage was no longer the happy union it once was prompted one woman to have an affair. Her husband, a diabetic, had been bedridden for fifteen years, but over the years he had become hostile, critical, and utterly without compassion. "For our twenty-fifth anniversary," she says, "the kids wanted to have a minister and renew our vows. I said I absolutely cannot do that. I was adamant. I think now I was starting to detach emotionally." She was infuriated that, although her children never offered to help her care for their father, they still expected her to maintain the facade of a happy couple. A man she worked with whose wife was bedridden from an accident had been asking her out for months, but she always refused. Then came the day of the anniversary party. "Everyone was upset that I didn't want to do wedding bells," she says. "So I went into the bedroom and closed the door. I picked up my portable phone and called this guy. I said, 'If that offer's still open for a movie, I'm ready.' We never made it to the movie." She feels, "God understands why I couldn't renew my wedding vows."

Despite all the reasons not to have an affair, the frustration of living as a "married widow or widower" may become too torturous. The connections we seek may not be sexual. One woman whose husband is in a nursing home with Parkinson's says, "I don't have any men friends, but I'd like to have. I'd just like someone who isn't a woman, someone to call in case the car's act-ing funny." Paul Kleffner's wife is in a nursing home with Alzheimer's, but he sees nothing wrong with seeking out female companionship; in fact, he considers it a necessity. "I don't talk to the children about this, because they're not too excited if I even take a woman out to dinner," he says. "But I have a few friends who are nice, attractive women, and women seem to like me. I feel most guilty when someone sees me with somebody else. But it doesn't bother me that much. I have to do it sometimes just to break this spell."

There are different kinds of intimacy, and an intimate friendship with a member of the opposite sex, one that allows the sharing of a wide range of thoughts and feelings, may be satisfying enough without becoming sexual. Just to have someone who gives us undivided attention, who doesn't fall over when we lean against him, who tells us how pretty we look in that new outfit—in short, all the things healthy people take for granted—would be heavenly. But first we must redefine our marriages and our roles in them.

After Don went to a nursing home, a counselor recommended I join a group for those who were "divorced, separated, and widowed." My husband objected. "You're not any of those," he said. But I was. I was separated from him by illness. I joined the support group, and it became a life-giving source of friendship and community with other single people. Their companionship—strictly platonic—got me through the first difficult years without Don. Support groups of various kinds can be places where relationships form, occasionally with the knowledge and approval of the sick partners.

For those who do find a sexual partner, the waters don't part after the affair starts. Entering into an affair, while it has its rewards, brings new questions and concerns. Trish, whose husband has had MS for twenty years, says, "I didn't go looking for it, it just found me. I have to admit, I fantasized about a relationship for a couple of years. Now, it's hard to deal with all the emotions I have, the wonderful feelings it gives you and the scary feelings it gives you. I felt cheated for so long, and got so tired of it. I don't like the word 'entitled,' but I'm going to use it anyway. I'm entitled to some type of life outside of work, caregiving, paying bills, taking the car to the repair shop, all that kind of stuff."

Another well spouse encouraged her. "She said, 'You could be diagnosed with cancer tomorrow. Then you'd look back and think, why didn't I get some enjoyment outside of this disease, outside of caregiving?'" Despite the exhilaration the relationship brings, she is terrified of her husband finding out. "I absolutely do not want to leave my husband, and I don't want a divorce. I still have a lot of love for him, even if it's not the love we started out with. I don't know for sure what I'm going to do."

Well spouses are often isolated because they devote so much time to caregiving, but a man I'll call George, whose wife has Parkinson's, met a woman in a support group whose husband was diabetic. "This woman wanted to have an affair with me, and her being interested in me did more for me than anything had for a long time. It changed my outlook on life," he says.

He began to see himself as someone who could make sexual choices. Although the woman lost her nerve before they had an affair, George was changed by knowing her. He subsequently met another woman with whom he became intimate. He is surprised at how little guilt he feels. "The Creator wants us to live to the fullest, in spite of marriage vows," he says. A woman, whose husband is a quad from an accident, voices a similar thought: "How can you cheat on somebody you're not having intimacy with?"

George sounds pretty certain of God's intentions for him, but the rest of us may wonder. Does God still expect us to keep the promises we made, or are we, in light of our changed circumstances, allowed some leeway? The irony that the same vows we thought guaranteed us a lifetime sexual partner now doom us to celibacy is not lost on us. We aren't in the marriages we thought we were entering when we said those vows, so how valid are the rules? Do they still apply?

My turning point came when I discovered a lump under my jaw. I thought it was a swollen gland, but after a year, it had not disappeared. An ear, nose, and throat specialist sent me for a CAT scan. I was able to deny the implications of the directive until I found myself inside the echoing metal tube. I had a moment of sheer terror. *Cancer!* I thought. *They're looking for cancer!*

The lump wasn't cancer but a cyst that had formed deep in my jaw. Although it required surgery, it was removed easily with no aftereffects.

Even so, I was shaken. What if it had been cancer? By then, Don had been in a nursing home three years as a hospice patient. When he went in, Dr. Shepard had told me he didn't think he would be alive after two years. Yet here we still were. Each wedding anniversary seemed a cruel mockery of the marriage we had once had. I realized that I had put my life on hold, waiting for him to die. Now I knew the clock was ticking for me too. All the loneliness, confusion, and anger I had been holding in for the past three years came pouring out when I met with my counselor. When I told her I was afraid I would die before I had ever lived, she said softly, "Chris, your husband is dying. But you don't have to die too." Her words pointed me in a new direction.

Medical crises are among the more dramatic wake-up calls. However, anniversaries, a friend's wedding, even a change of season can have the same effect. We're aware, as never before, of the deserts of vast eternity all around us.

Make no mistake, having an affair, for most of us, is not

simply about scratching an itch. The reason the decision feels so momentous is that it requires us to redefine our marriage vows and, along with those, our lifelong beliefs about marriage. It requires that we ask the biggest question of all: What's right and wrong? Most societies strongly condemn sex outside of marriage. Violating that rule, which may have been a deeply held rule of our own, feels terrifying. Before we can act, however, we must acknowledge the kind of marriages we have now. Before the illness, we thought of ourselves as a twosome, a partnership, a couple. Admitting that the "we-ness" of our union is going, or gone, that now our needs are different from our spouse's, can be a painful awakening. Deciding to be sexual with someone else means deciding in favor of our own needs. It can feel like the ultimate betrayal of our partners.

The well spouse experience needs a language, and hasn't evolved one yet. The word "affair" sounds too frivolous, and too illicit, for what becomes, for many, a life-saving, and marriage-saving, decision. In order to see our marriages clearly, and thus empower ourselves, we must redefine the "terminology of fidelity" to fit our lives—our real lives, not the ones other people, and maybe our own spouses, think we are living. Being able to name what's missing helps us decide whether an extramarital relationship would be the answer. Then, "What's holding me back?" is the next question we need to answer. Sometimes we discover that we ourselves, not our children, our neighbors, or our church, are the biggest obstacle. What I needed when I sought out a "lover," another word that doesn't sound right, was less the sex than someone to hold me, to ease the aching sadness of watching my beloved husband die.

The guilt that may accompany an affair can certainly mitigate, and maybe eliminate, the pleasure it brings. A man who is having an affair put words to the moral quandary he feels. "Are these bits and pieces of happiness yet another insidious form of temptation from the Dark One? Or are these short interludes of bliss and the ensuing hopeful dreams partial compensation from God for countless days of steadfast care? A case can be made either way."

Deciding whether to have an affair took me years. Since Don had gone to the nursing home, I had been unbearably lonely. Yet I couldn't act. I had been raised Catholic and educated in Catholic schools, the quintessential "good Catholic girl." Don and I had exchanged rings in a nuptial mass, and attended mass regularly. Of all the things I had imagined myself doing over the course of a lifetime, seeking out another man while I was still married was never one of them. To complicate things, I lived in a small town, with two impressionable preteens at home. I also wondered, guiltily, if I was justified in seeking sexual companionship if I was still able to have sex, though very limited sex, with my husband. But I was starting to resent Don's expectation that I pretend our marriage was normal, when it was anything but. The last thing I wanted was to hate him for being sick. It seemed logical to look for a pressure valve.

Looking for someone to advise me, I visited a distant relative whose first husband had died after a long illness. "Look at yourself," she urged. "It's not as if your husband is able to do things with you and travel with you, and can't think of what to buy you next. You need to do some things that make *you* happy." Still I held off . . . tempted but afraid.

I was caught off guard when my counselor suggested, "Why not have both, then?" I had been thinking only of what an affair might take away from my husband, never of what it might bring him. For the first time I wondered if an affair could enrich his life too, by making me more fulfilled. Maybe I could even ask Don how he felt.

This was tender new ground. How could I let Don know I wanted men friends in my life without hurting him deeply? One woman whose husband has MS says, "One time he said to me, 'I wish I was dead so you could get on with your life.' When he said that, I thought about asking whether he would consider letting me get on with just a small little segment of my life at this time— like an affair. But unless he brings it up, I would not bring it up, because I absolutely don't think he could understand."

Sometimes a sick partner encourages an affair, at least in theory. Roy Layton says his wife, Donna, "claimed she was agreeable to me finding some pleasure somewhere else. But when it was an actual fact, she wasn't able to have the same attitude she expounded before. She was angry and hurt." Gaelene Farrell's thirty-two-year-old husband, Wayne, is on dialysis because of diabetes. She is twenty-seven. She says, "When he first started having severe problems, he said, 'Let's divorce so you can go on with your life.'" But, she adds, "I don't think he means it."

I began to broach the subject tentatively with Don, who struggled with the question during many sessions with his counselor. Eventually, in a "letting go" session mediated by her, he agreed, with the stipulation, "as long as I don't have to hear about it." We could never have negotiated so great a leap if this therapist had not been Catholic too. Both of us liked and trusted her, but she had formed a special bond with Don. She reminded us of the love and trust we had developed over the course of the illness, and encouraged us to depend on those bonds now to always bring us back to each other.

After that day, I felt lighter, more as if being "faithful" was a choice I was making rather than a condition placed on me. I told myself that Don couldn't live forever as sick as he was, and I could wait. The months passed.

August 19, 1992, was our twentieth wedding anniversary, and

I arranged for our parish priest to come to the nursing home. After blessing us, Father Patton asked Don if he wanted to renew our wedding vows. Don hesitated a moment, then shook his head. He offered me a gift only he could give me, my freedom. I understood that he meant what he had said before.

Before going any further, I talked to my children individually, and told them that their dad had agreed to let me have men friends. Tim immediately approved of the idea. Meg had misgivings, but I explained that these friendships would not affect my love or caring for Don, her, or Tim.

A few months later, I met a man at a temporary job who was from out of town, which made discretion easier. He was divorcing, and I like to think that our affair, which lasted about a year, helped us both through a difficult time.

Maybe Don was able to let me go because, by then, he had given up almost everything except his life. And maybe, if our doctor had not given him a limited time to live, he would not have been able to. Maybe I wouldn't have asked him. I'll never know. I know that I was awed by the trust he had in me, which brought us closer than ever. The affair awakened me to the profound love I had for Don. My lover, while offering me physical release, couldn't offer me anything like the emotional intimacy I had with my husband. I brought a new sexual energy to our bed, because I recognized that making love with him was infinitely more meaningful than an afternoon with my athletic lover. I was overwhelmed and humbled by the discovery that having an affair did not mean that Don suffered. Paradoxically, pursuing my own path brought rewards to both of us.

Nurturing ourselves can make us better partners to our sick mates, because we have more to give them. Just as I had to acknowledge that my husband and I were separated, not by choice but by circumstances, I had to redefine faithful and unfaithful. I know that having an affair was not being unfaithful. Instead, it made me more faithful.

Five years after Don's death, I still feel ambivalent about that time. I believe my affair strengthened my marriage, and while I don't regret it, I regret that it was necessary. I honored Don's wishes by not telling him about it, but if I'm honest with myself, I know he probably suspected something. Like so many decisions I made during his life, this one didn't feel quite right—or quite wrong. But then, no decision ever had that good, clean sense of "having done the right thing." I am sure of this: Whether we decide to risk an affair or not, we've stayed in our marriages in order to make our partners' lives bearable. Finding some happiness for ourselves doesn't have to take anything away from our partners. It may bring unexpected gifts to both of us.

# 5. Money:
# Never Enough

 In the spring of 1986, the future looked bright for the Herndon family of Summersville, West Virginia. David had a good job as a coal miner and his wife, Kay, recently recertified as a teacher, was going to start teaching fifth grade in the fall. With their three children in high school and planning on college, the Herndons would need both incomes. "We were about to go from $40,000 to $70,000 a year," says David.

Then Kay began to have problems with balance. Initially, doctors thought she had MS, but a year later, when an MRI showed cerebellar degeneration, the diagnosis was changed to Parkinson's disease. Soon Kay began having problems with incontinence, then with speaking and swallowing. Within two years, she needed twenty-four-hour attention. Looking back, David realizes, "We would have been better off financially if we had divorced. But it wasn't a choice I wanted to make." David's health insurance paid for only four hours a day, forty days a year, of home care. Despite his $38,000 a year salary, Kay's care was draining them. They weren't poor enough for Medicaid, and local health services provided only what insurance would cover.

David's employer graciously agreed to lay him off so that he could collect $900 a month unemployment and care for his wife full-time. A Social Security lawyer he consulted told him the same things he had heard earlier from county health services: Kay, at forty-three, was too young for Medicare and hadn't paid into Social Security. The Herndons were about to "fall through the cracks of the system," the lawyer said. The only choice seemed to be spiraling down into poverty so that Kay would qualify for Medicaid. That, at least, was easy. By December 1988, they had spent their savings and investments and were well on their way. By then, Kay could have entered a nursing home and Medicaid would have paid for her care. But the Herndons couldn't face the idea of living apart. In spite of her physical problems, Kay's mind was good. She and David still loved each other. They still had one asset, their home, but if they were to afford Kay's medical necessities and care—she needed a gastric tube implanted surgically because she could no longer swallow, as well as an indwelling catheter—they would have to give that up too. They moved to a handicapped-accessible apartment, and David became the resident manager, earning about $200 a month. With Kay's SSI (a government program for the medically needy poor) of $407 a month, they resigned themselves "to being poor and staying that way." Kay died in 1992, but David, permanently disillusioned by what he went through, does volunteer work and stays poor. For him, the American Dream is a hoax. "Our community helped us tremendously with volunteer help," he says. "But our government, in terms of its being able to help families with long-term chronic illness, was a failure. I still don't see any legislation that's designed to help families stay together.

A national health care program should be the number one
priority."

Not all well spouse stories are as haunting as David's, but his
is not unique. No one is ever prepared to deal with the costs of a
catastrophic illness. Sometimes, as in David's case, all the worst
"what ifs" come true. Barbara Beachman couldn't afford respite
care for her husband, and became so exhausted she ended up running away from home. John Hardin lost his farm because of his
wife Nancy's illness, a lupus-like condition that caused seizures.
Nancy's illness put them on welfare—that was the only way they
could qualify for medical assistance in 1982. "Now, they have a
thing called a medical assistance waiver [a result of the Spousal
Impoverishment Act, passed in 1989]," says John. "You have to
be income-eligible, from the sick person's perspective, but I can
make as much money as I can make, and it doesn't limit Nancy's
benefits." Welfare, he says, was demoralizing because "when you
most want to, you can't go to work. You just sit home and get
depressed." Unfortunately, the law changed too late to help the
Herndons.

When her husband, Pat, began needing operations for
chronic pancreatitis, Donna Keefe says they had to scale down
financially, but they have landed on their feet. "Where we lived
before we had a house, and a yard, and a garage, and all the toys
people have. And we lost that." The house sale, while heart-
breaking for Donna, enabled them to pay their bills and buy a
trailer. Now that Pat is on disability and retirement, says Donna,
"we're not hurting for money at all." One possession she can't
bring herself to sell is their camper, a reminder of the fun they
used to have at a nearby lake. "It's a part of the past I can't part
with yet," she says.

With an illness whose onset is sudden and serious, the money woes are equally so. Jim Maxwell's doctor prescribed steroid tablets to help his MS, but they cost $1.20 apiece, and he needed twenty-five a day—a fearsome expense for a young couple just starting to find their financial feet. Diane started selling possessions to afford the payments on their new truck. She was working for low wages at a day care center, and with Jim unable to run the refrigeration business they had just bought, they were desperate for cash. Diane sold the land they had hoped to build on and prayed the pills would alleviate Jim's one-sided paralysis. Still, "it was eight months before we saw some changes in him," she says. They were fortunate that, eventually, Jim entered an eighteen-year remission.

Money is the foundation we build our dreams on; when the money fades, dreams fade too. Gaelene Farrell says wistfully, "I thought we would be a normal couple, that we'd get married and buy a house. I thought we'd have a few financial problems, but that we'd be like most couples, going on trips together, buying nice clothes. Financial worries are one of the hardest things about this." When illness hits in the middle years, retirement plans are shelved. Either we have to keep working to pay medical bills, or there's nothing to retire to. Mark Johannes says, "When I retired, I was very jealous, very envious of the other guys, my peers, who I knew would be retiring to unlimited fishing trips or driving trips all over the country, with not a care in the world, and all this money to spend on anything they wanted. Where, in the last ten years, we've spent $40,000 on remodeling and medical expenses, just for this disease."

Those whose income keeps them even with expenses are lucky, and they know it. Eugenia Staerker, a college administrator, says, "I have a position that pays me enough money to make my bills. I have a medical prescription plan, and if I didn't have that, I'd be hard pressed. One of Ray's drugs is one hundred forty-seven dollars."

It's axiomatic among well spouses that women become caregivers, but men, with their higher earning capacity, hire caregivers. One man whose wife has Alzheimer's works as a lawyer for a publishing company. He says, "I'm pretty free to come and go. I have twenty-four-hour care for my wife. I earn a good income, and I can afford it." He says that he loves his work, and has adjusted fairly well to his wife's problems because work is his escape. He exemplifies one wife's statement that "money makes the difference in how well spouses cope."

But even a spouse who earns a good salary will feel pinched if his partner needs round-the-clock care. An attorney whose wife has had a series of strokes says, "The high emotional and physical energy required for me to continue the stressful life of a busy attorney slowly receded in inverse order to the advance of her illness. I slowly spun down and my earning abilities did too. The result for me is a large loss of income. I am sixty-one years old, and should be at the top of my earning years, and should reasonably expect to have another ten solid years ahead. Instead, I am semi-retired and practicing law out of my house in order to be the primary caregiver so we can save money."

Starting with the myelogram, I began to grasp the financial implications of having a husband with an incurable illness. I was shocked when we began to price equipment. It seemed to me that in a caring society, anyone with the bad luck to be stricken with a bad illness should be given whatever he needed, delivered the same day, gift-wrapped, with the condolences of the community. No such benevolent agency existed then or now, of course. I soon realized that multiple sclerosis might impoverish us not just in human terms, but in monetary ones as well.

We were lucky to be covered by health insurance through Don's job, because it covered 80 percent of the drugs he needed. That left us paying 20 percent, but at least it wasn't 100 percent. Equipment was covered, too, but the insurance company required letters from our doctor explaining that each purchase was "medically necessary," so we usually had to buy first, then wait to be reimbursed. We rarely got an argument, but we were always waiting for the check. Were they really afraid we'd go on a spending spree buying medical equipment we could hardly stand the sight of? ("Whee, Honey, let's buy three portable commodes instead of one!") I was appalled that a few pieces of plastic and steel could cost hundreds of dollars. A "feeding machine" consisting of some metal tubing and a leather sling cost $1,500.

Medical equipment companies seemed determined to take advantage of those who could afford it least. If middle-income people like Don and me thought this stuff was expensive, how on earth did poor people afford it? The lawyer who works out of his home to take care of his wife says, "There is no bargaining power for the desperate souls who are forced to buy the merchandise. People have no choice. Needing catheter bags or underpads or adult diapers for incontinence isn't like trying to decide whether to buy a new gas grill for your patio. This 'Gotcha Business' of medical equipment and supplies is tailored for reimbursement out of the deep pockets of medical insurance companies, and not from people who have holes in their pockets with little or no medical insurance or high deductibles." Of course, even if insurance pays, we all pay for such gouging eventually in higher premiums and deductibles.

With most of the household money going toward illness, less is left for discretionary spending. What's left can make or break the marriage. For women, a husband's money can be an important factor in their decision to stay married. In spite of equal employment laws, women still straggle far behind men in earning capacity. With their lives severely circumscribed, having money allows well wives the vacations, gym memberships, clothes, and jewelry that offset the sacrifices. Bette Allbright's husband, Jim, got MS in 1973, and initially, she had no doubts about staying with him. Her resolve weakened as he became increasingly crippled. He was often short-tempered with their two girls, and with her too. Could she stay with him? Should she? By her thirtieth birthday, seven years into the MS, she set herself a deadline of her thirty-fifth birthday. Five years, she reasoned, ought to be enough time to decide. "Turning thirty didn't bother me," she says. "But what bothered me was having to spend more time with the situation getting worse."

When the day came and Jim didn't mention the occasion, she went to a jewelry store and bought herself an extravagant diamond ring. Flashing the ring at him, she warned, "Don't ever forget my birthday again." He was unfazed by the money she had spent, and she realized that he was giving her tacit approval to spend what she needed on herself. She decided to stay in her marriage. Today, twenty-four years after Jim's diagnosis, she feels she has too many years invested to bail out.

Another woman, whose husband's kidney disease made him increasingly bad-tempered and controlling, says, "I had no way to support myself in the way I was accustomed to living, and that was important to me. But my husband had a profitable manufacturing business, so I had as much money as I wanted. And I stayed." More than one wife said she hung on for the life insurance policies.

In the United States, social status depends on one's ability to acquire money and possessions. Predictably, a high-energy, take-no-prisoners executive, feared and admired in the workplace, and used to earning in the six figures, doesn't adapt well to the helplessness of chronic illness. Americans define themselves in terms of employment, and someone who isn't employed has lost both his work identity and his earning power—two big losses. A woman whose husband has severe angina says that, when she married him at twenty-two, "he was never easy, but he was wonderful and caring, and the best friend you'd want to have in the world." Those traits were what made her marry him. Formerly the CEO of a medium-sized corporation, he hasn't made peace with the early retirement his heart disease has forced him into. "He's controlling, always has been, and thinks very little of himself, which is reflected in the way he directs other people. He thinks since he has this physical disability, he's less of a person. I guess it makes him feel better to take others down. He feels a little better when he's criticizing someone else," she says. Unfortunately, his criticism is often directed at her, "because," she says, "I'm here more than anyone."

The person who earns more in a marriage often gets a bigger say, not only in how the money is spent, but in other decisions too. When the primary wage earner, usually the husband, gets sick, his self-esteem is improved if he stays involved in making household money decisions. Sharing such decisions helps a husband and wife maintain the power balance, and reassures the sick partner that he is still a viable part of the couple. Donna Keefe says that she and her husband, Pat, "think alike on money matters." She puts the wages from her job as a housekeeper at an adolescent treatment center in the checkbook, and Pat pays the bills—a chore she hates. Neither likes debt, and they are careful to pay off their credit card balances promptly. Nevertheless, when Pat was in the hospital for surgery, Donna found that even though she didn't like paying the bills, she liked controlling the checkbook. She didn't want to give it back to Pat after he recuperated, but she did. She also asks his permission to use their credit cards to buy Christmas gifts. "I could have used them anyway," she says. "But I ask. I want Pat to be important and make decisions. He hasn't got that much left, because he can't work." Encouraging a sick spouse to do the things he still can do makes for less resentment.

Barbara Drucker's husband, David, has had MS for twenty years, but they continue to share financial responsibilities as they've always done. "David was a dentist," she says, "and he's always been an investor. So we're pretty financially secure, and we really don't have money problems." Barbara is in charge of paying the bills and making sure there's money in the checking account. "I like to know where the money's going," she says. "David is still the chief investor, and I hope he's doing a good job. He seems to be, and I kind of watch that he doesn't make any wild and crazy decisions." Wives may take a policy of watchful waiting to make sure husbands don't start throwing money away—although they do sometimes. Carly, whose husband, Mike, has scleroderma, has tried without success to talk him out of wrongheaded financial decisions. "I don't think the route for me is to march in to an attorney with my power of attorney and demand psychological testing," she says. "I'm going to some local attorney, and he's going to get some Madison Avenue attorneys, and that's a fair fight? He's a master of manipulation, and believe me, he could cry any story he wants and they'd believe him." She sees his overly optimistic thinking as a denial mechanism. "I consider it a no-win situation, and I'm not going to fight it," she says. Another wife, who worked all day while her husband stayed home, didn't realize his bipolar disorder, a mental illness characterized by periods of euphoria alternating with depression, made him easy prey for fraudulent telephone sales. "When he was in an 'up mood,' he believed anything they told him," she says. After he died, she was stunned to find he'd lost thousands of dollars.

She was able to reclaim some after threatening the companies with lawsuits; the rest is gone. "I've just had to put it behind me," she says.

For Debbie Lang, her husband Dan's spending went haywire because of his Parkinson's dementia, and after he went to a nursing home, she was left with a garage full of electronic gadgets he bought for his experiments, and other grownup toys. She was relieved at regaining control of the money and she overspent. "At first, it was like, you're gone, so now my kids are going to get what they need. It felt like revenge." When she realized her bills weren't getting paid, she went back to more moderate spending. With Dan safely confined, she has opened a day care center in her home.

Keeping a job if you have one and getting one if you don't is a sanity-saver, even if the paycheck isn't lavish. Having a job helps nurture an identity separate from the illness, and is worth the effort. Natalie is a high school guidance counselor. She says, "I need there to be a part of me separate from Dennis. I need there to be a part that can grow, and not be attached to sickness all the time. And professionally, I'm separate. I'm good at what I do and like what I do." Joan Fanti had started a pet-grooming business a few months before her husband fell from a gravel sifter at work and became a quad. "I kept it going," she says of her business. "It was probably the only thing that kept me sane."

Money worries add to the general anxiety in our households—as if there wasn't enough already. Unexpected equipment failures and changes in a spouse's condition bring more expenses. I found it impossible not to obsess about money, but was ashamed when I did. After all, what was more important than Don's ability to function in his narrowing world? He deserved anything that would make his life livable. But I couldn't help worrying. How would we pay for the endless parade of equipment, drugs, and health aides we would need? Even with insurance that paid most of the "reasonable and customary" costs, 20 percent could add up to a lot of money. And what about the costs insurance wouldn't pay, but Don might want to try—bee venom, acupuncture, magnets? Where incurable illness is concerned, quacks abound. Dr. Shepard warned us against spending money searching out bogus treatments. "There's no cure for MS," he said flatly. Thank goodness my sensible husband listened. *But, I wondered, what if, as he gets worse, he wants to travel the world? What if he needs an operation, or two, or five? If he wants something expensive, how can I refuse him?*

For Don and me, equipment and drugs, covered by insurance, weren't a problem. Home health care was, and with an illness like MS, he needed more and more of it. Here, our luck ran out. Private insurance companies follow Medicare's lead in determining what they cover, and frequently, if Medicare won't pay, they won't either. Don and I ran up a big balance with a local home health agency, which allowed us to pay a little each month. When it came to getting home help, living in a small community was both good and bad. The cost of an aide was reasonable at $9 an hour, but Helena had only two home health agencies, neither of which had many employees. Don had lost weight over the course of the illness, but he was still too heavy, at 180 pounds, for most women, and a lot of men, to lift. Some came once and refused to return, afraid of straining their backs or irritating an old injury. At that time, we didn't have a Hoyer lift. I was so grateful to be getting any help, I didn't begrudge these people the money they were paid—barely $5 an hour after the agency took its cut, with no reimbursement for mileage, even though they used their own cars. But it was the most menial of menial work, and in many cases, it attracted people who couldn't do anything else. Some, instead of quitting, just didn't show up. Some had car problems that made them late or absent. Some had attitude problems. I was never sure who would walk through the door each day, with access to my home, my children, and my husband's most intimate care. Some were gems, and we missed them when they left. But we didn't have the money to entice them to stay, so we took what came.

Money considerations shouldn't taint a decision as emotional as putting a spouse in a nursing home, but of course they do. Our insurance company, in spite of letters from us and our doctor, stubbornly refused to pay for home health care, but our interpretation of Don's employee benefits led us to think they might cover skilled nursing care. Our options were few. The costs of home health care were getting to be several hundred dollars a month. Finding someone to live in might have worked if our house had been bigger, but all the bedrooms were full. We had run out of choices.

I remember the stretch between his admission in September and the January day the letter came from the insurance company as one of the most terrifying periods of my life. I jumped when the phone rang, afraid it might be bad news. Every afternoon I approached the mailbox as if it might contain a nest of cobras. The bills came regularly from the nursing home in breathtaking amounts, $2,200, $2,300; soon a stamp at the bottom scolded that the account was past due. I consulted a lawyer on his interpretation of Don's employee benefits (he felt the insurance company might pay), and asked him about divorcing Don to make him poor enough for Medicaid (Don was earning most of the money, so that was probably not a good idea). Of all the nightmares I could conjure up, that was the worst, to have to renounce the vows I believed in and the husband I loved in order to get his care paid for. But if the insurance company refused us, I might have no alternative. One woman who got a legal separation from her young husband, with severe MS, in order to get Medicaid, told me, "I felt so sleazy, like I was ripping off the system." But she felt she had no alternative. She could either keep her husband in the nursing home or a roof over herself and her young son, but she couldn't do both.

Divorcing to get money is a repugnant idea for most of us, to be used only as a last resort. Jim Russell says of his wife, Hannah, "I can't divorce her. It would be a friendly divorce, obviously, to get her Medicaid. But divorce is a lawsuit, it isn't friendly. I mean, OK, we wink, but it's a lawsuit, and the state appoints an attorney, and his job is to make sure she gets everything she's entitled to."

However, since the Spousal Impoverishment Act of 1989, the amount of money and assets a well spouse can keep and still allow a partner to qualify for Medicaid has increased. These amounts vary from state to state, but in Montana a well spouse can keep half the cash and assets owned by the couple, no matter which partner earned them, up to $90,000, in addition to the home he or she lives in. Because a well spouse can keep so much more money now, having to divorce to collect Medicaid is less likely to be necessary. Many couples, if the spouse needs care long enough, will have to apply for Medicaid—there's simply no other way to afford the $30,000 a year most nursing homes cost.

For those who have accumulated considerable savings, spending down in order to qualify for Medicaid feels all wrong. Jim Russell's successful computer business has allowed him to acquire substantial savings, but those may have to go. "There's something called 'spousal refusal' in New York State, and that's the approach we're thinking of taking," he says. "The spend-down I'd be allowed to keep is $75,000 plus the house and the car. All the rest would have to be spent. We're talking about taking a couple of hand grenades and dropping them down into our future." He is consulting elder-law attorneys to make sure that's the only choice before he decides what to do.

The process of trying to qualify a spouse can be grueling, irrespective of the outcome. "This isn't just hard emotionally," says a woman whose husband has Parkinson's. "It's all the legal things. It took two years to get him on Medi-Cal [California's equivalent of Medicaid]. It would have cost me four thousand dollars a month for his nursing home. I had to go to court. I got an attorney, and it cost me fifteen thousand dollars. I had to get a court order so that I can sign for him. I still pay eight hundred dollars a month. It's not a hardship. Well, let me amend that. It could be worse." But she never stops worrying. "I wasn't aware that every year they do a redetermination of benefits. You bet I worry about that. If you don't fill in the forms exactly right, they take the Medi-Cal away. I pay someone to help me with that, because God forbid I should do something wrong."

Bob Keller's wife, Ellen, is in a nursing home with Alzheimer's, and he had to spend down to qualify Ellen for help. It didn't take long, with the costs of her care running $3,600 per month. After he was down to $68,000, plus his house, he was allowed simply to turn over her Social Security check to the nursing home, keeping $40 a month for her personal items. The government pays the rest. More than anything, he says, he resents "being under the thumb of the government." He says, "I've never been unemployed in my life, so I've never drawn unemployment. So, to me, it's putting your hand out for something you really shouldn't have to." If he goes on a trip or buys a new car, he must report those expenditures.

The unfairness of having to beg after a lifetime of paying into the system angers the woman whose husband is on Medi-Cal too.

"My lawyer wrote a letter to the judge, how rich people have all kinds of loopholes, and here's a man that has worked hard all his life, and paid all his taxes, and everything. He didn't retire until he was seventy."

If money were only currency, writing checks to a nursing home wouldn't sting so much. But money represents dreams and hopes and pleasures deferred in favor of a shared future: travel, a vacation home, a luxury car, a retirement business—all of which you'd planned to enjoy with a loved partner. Margy Kleinerman says, "Joe's retirement check covers the nursing home, and I have my retirement check. But when I make out the check for the nursing home, although he's in an excellent one, and you get what you pay for, then comes the resentful part. We're in the middle, as are hundreds of people, thousands of people." Paying the nursing home is a bitter reminder that your spouse won't be able to do any of the things you'd planned.

Instead of spending down assets to obtain Medicaid, some spouses give everything away to their children in arrangements known as irrevocable trusts, but the giveaway must occur thirty months before the sick spouse can get Medicaid—and your children must be absolutely trustworthy. If they spend the money or lose it in a divorce, you have no recourse against them. This option has worked well for Paul Kleffner, whose wife, Thelma, is in a nursing home that costs $3,000 a month. "I'm getting by fine now," he says. "Everything is in a trust. I'm really a pauper, you might say, and dependent on my children. They don't give me money, except the money in the trust I'm entitled to. They allow me to live off the trust." He says he got good advice from two attorneys as well as a CPA.

The two best rules for making sure you won't lose everything are to get expert advice and to plan ahead. "You have approximately five years from the time you're diagnosed to the time you generally quit working," says Laura Cooper, a life planning and legal consultant for the National MS Society. "The one way that people's lives are wrecked, more often than not, is financially," she says. "Soon after a diagnosis, people should engage in a very thorough life plan, using an elder lawyer. This person can send them off to a financial planner, and these lawyers also have knowledge and information about housing and Medicaid and Medicare and Social Security, all of those things. They should be able to read people's health and life and disability plans and know where the gaps are." Since laws differ from state to state, you need a lawyer versed in your state's laws. Your state bar association can refer you to an elder-law attorney, and a national association of elder lawyers is listed in the back of this book.

For most of us, talking about financial matters with a spouse, especially when it comes to affording a nursing home for them, is touchy, but doing so in advance is much better than having decisions made for you after it's too late. One wife says, "When I bring it up, he says, 'Oh, you're getting ready to put me in a nursing home.' I say, 'I'm not getting ready, but it's a possibility. It's something we have to plan for.'" She has already looked into the laws in her state, a wise course of action. "Mine is a really bad state to live in that way," she says. On the other hand, a neighboring state is much more liberal in what it will allow a well spouse to keep, and she is considering moving if and when the time comes. "It's a definite possibility," she says.

Don't overlook any possible sources of financial help. Our county had a vocational rehabilitation fund that helped purchase equipment deemed necessary to keep someone employed, and helped us buy a wheelchair for Don. Service clubs in your area may help you buy equipment. One woman said her local MS chapter maintained a respite fund so that well spouses could get away occasionally. A young person stricken with an illness hasn't held as many jobs as an older person, but it may be worthwhile to ask previous employers whether health insurance or disability policies still exist. Don't forget military disability if your spouse is a veteran. After Hank's head injury, Hilde felt panicky when she looked ahead. "All of a sudden, there was the breadwinner, gone," she says. Hank had been a teacher, and hadn't paid into Social Security, so he wasn't eligible for benefits. Her minimum wage job and Hank's teacher's retirement amounted to only a fraction of the income they would need. Hank's boss came to her rescue by persuading her to apply for a 100 percent military disability for Hank. He argued that if Hank's leg hadn't been partly paralyzed from a service-related injury, he might have been able to brake sooner, and his injuries wouldn't have been so severe. To Hilde's amazement, the application came back approved—only a week before Hank was to be discharged from the rehab unit. Now they are able to live on his veteran's benefits.

If there's any possibility your insurance will cover the cost of a nursing home, persevere in persuading them. An attorney letter, if you think they're wavering or giving you the runaround, is a good incentive. I think I kissed the mailbox, and everyone else in sight, the day our insurance company notified us they would cover Don's care because he was in a skilled facility. We may have had an edge because he worked in the insurance business, although the employee health insurance was contracted to a different insurance company. Our family doctor, who diagnosed Don, went to bat for us again and again to help us get benefits from different sources. Thanks to him, Don was approved for Social Security disability the first time we applied, a process that sometimes takes several tries. As early in the illness as possible, look for medical professionals you can trust—then stay with them. Building a relationship with one physician can be very valuable, not just because your spouse needs good medical care, but because a physician's word is rarely questioned by insurance companies and government agencies. The right letter from the right doctor at the right time can work wonders. A family physician who has known and treated your whole family over the course of the illness may be more likely than a specialist to go the extra mile because he or she has seen all of you struggle with the human costs of the illness.

# 6. Anger: Slaves in the Cellar

Constant loss means constant anger; only the levels fluctuate. Frustration is its mildest form, and blinding rage its most dangerous, but it's always simmering below the surface, threatening to erupt. We feel cheated out of so much; just the sight of a couple walking arm in arm down a street is enough to turn a promising day into a black funk.

Hollywood perpetuates the myth that caregiving is satisfying, and that illness brings out the best in families, especially the sick person. Well spouses sit in the audience and think, who are these people? Of course, Hollywood thinks death is beautiful, so illness must be, too. Remember Ali MacGraw's dying in *Love Story?* More recently, I had to stifle a giggle when in *The English Patient* Ralph Fiennes's character goes back to the desert to retrieve his dead mistress. Although she's been dead for weeks in the baking heat, and should be the consistency of a potato chip, he is nevertheless able to drape her limply over his arms. Her skin is moist and rosy, eyes peacefully closed. In an article for the *New York*

*Times Magazine*, former well spouse Jane Bendetson took on the movie *Marvin's Room*, saying: "I just don't know anyone like the character Diane Keaton played." This character "smiles beatifically" when awakened at 3:00 A.M., and turns down her sister's offer of help. "I'm used to it after so many years," says the Keaton character. Bendetson continues, "She speaks of the love that she receives from her bedridden father and senile aunt, but I hear very different reactions from caregivers: anguish, as love, hope, expectations, and life itself erode in tiny increments."

Don was in a nursing home when I saw *My Life*, with Michael Keaton. Diagnosed with terminal cancer, the Keaton character uses the time he has left to heal old rifts with his family, and thus dies surrounded by loving faces. But the character that really baffled me was Keaton's long-suffering wife, played by Nicole Kidman. Nowhere was there a sense that this woman felt wronged by the fact that her young husband was dying. Always reasonable and soft-spoken, she bore no resemblance to any well spouse I've ever known. I waited for the scene when she would fly into a crockery-throwing rage, or smack their excruciatingly adorable child for whining, or yell at a home health aide for being late (Oops, I forgot. No outside help for this efficient little family), or castigate Blue Cross for not covering Michael's Depends. Maybe she would even tell Keaton she hated him for dying and leaving her alone. But no. She remained colorless to the end, never showing any kind of emotion besides a subdued sadness. There's plenty of sadness in our lives, to be sure. But for most of us, anger is the monster that, to our dismay, colors our days and nights in shades of red.

It's tempting to dismiss these movies as being just entertainment. Unfortunately, the myths they promote are as contagious as they are insidious. People believe movie stereotypes, and expect well spouses to be ever-patient, ever-accommodating, self-reliant saints, like the ones they see on the silver screen. That expectation is unfair enough. But if well spouses believe the stereotypes, too, and start blaming themselves for not smiling as they empty a bedpan at 3:00 A.M., or not being a combination caregiver and single parent and job-holder with the serenity of Nicole Kidman, an already difficult situation becomes impossible.

Well spouses have so many things to be angry about that it's hard to pick a target. The steady loss of a partner's abilities—and the drip-drip-drip way it happens. The obtuseness and callousness of professionals. The incomprehension of the rest of the world. The gradual falling away of friends and family, as those we thought we could depend on, who we were certain would be with us through thick and thin, simply can't go the distance.

"Others owe us what we think they will give us. We must forgive them this debt," wrote Simone Weil. The wisdom of that statement stuck in Janelle's throat like a bone. That she would have to forgive those who should have been there for them, her husband's own brother and his wife, after the pummeling they had taken with Mark's MS, was a blow she hadn't anticipated. When she and Mark, who was then healthy, moved to the town where his brother lived, Steve and Joan Radley (not their real names), were delighted. Janelle was pleased that Steve and Joan dropped in often just to visit—sometimes alone, sometimes together. The Radleys loved to play bridge, and taught Mark and Janelle how to play. The two couples often got together for card games that lasted late into the evening. Mark and Steve's banter about their childhoods got them all laughing. Janelle and Mark had never had such a close couple friendship, having gone through the "love-him/can't-stand-her, love-her/can't-stand-him" experience before in their marriage. The fact that Mark and

Steve were brothers was the icing on the cake for Janelle, making their relationship even more special—more permanent, she believed.

Then Mark was diagnosed with MS, and the closeness began to erode. The drop-in visits became fewer. Mark waited a long weekend for Steve to call and invite him hunting, as he had done in the past. The call never came, and Janelle's heart ached for her husband. She wondered if it was because Mark's balance was getting unpredictable, and Steve didn't want the worry. Mark soon needed a wheelchair, and when they did visit the Radleys, it was difficult for Steve to get him up and down their front steps. Steve changed jobs, and the Radleys began to socialize more with people in his office. Mark and Janelle weren't included in their gatherings. Sometimes Joan, without Steve, dropped by, but her brief visits only reminded Janelle of the hours they had spent playing cards, eating together, or just visiting. *We need you more than ever*, she thought. *Especially Mark.* But she could never bring up the subject with Steve. After all, he was Mark's responsibility. She complained to Mark about his brother's withdrawal, but she hated to interfere. What if she caused family problems by speaking out? And Mark never wanted to bring it up. *Maybe it doesn't bother him*, thought Janelle. But it bothered her.

Mark had been in a wheelchair for eight years when he fell in the bathroom and hit his head on the sink. His head injury turned out to be serious. He was in a coma for a few days, and emerged with permanent brain damage. Janelle felt the world was ending. Mark's MS had been bad enough, but his cognitive functioning had been good. Now his short-term memory was gone, and he couldn't follow a simple conversation.

Mark was still in the hospital for his birthday, but Steve didn't visit—not even to pop his head in. After Janelle brought him home the Radleys dropped by with presents, but the gesture, to Janelle, was too little and way too late. She excused herself and went to the kitchen, where she furiously began to throw dirty dishes in the dishwasher. *Can't you see it's too late now?* she wanted to scream at them. *Where were you when we needed you?* She knew that Mark would probably have to go to a nursing home soon, and all hope of regaining the friendship they had known, a dream she had never given up on, was gone. Joan, noticing Janelle's coldness, called later to ask her what was wrong. All the anger Janelle had pushed down for so long erupted. She told Joan how their withdrawal had hurt her and Mark, and how angry she was now that they could never be close like they were. "The sicker Mark got, the less we saw of you!" she cried. Joan wept. She admitted that it had been Steve's reluctance to have Mark around that had set their course. Janelle was outraged.

Her counselor, usually helpful, made her feel worse. "Well, maybe if this couple, the Radleys, couldn't be there for you, another couple could have," she offered sweetly. Janelle wanted to reach over and grab her by the throat. *Sure,* she thought bitterly. *After a day that took everything we had to cope with this horrible illness, Mark and I couldn't wait to bring out the bubbly and engage in scintillating conversation.* The woman hadn't a clue. Making couple friends was tricky even for healthy couples, who could go places and do things. Where would the hours have come from to cultivate the kinds of deep friendships this woman had in mind? Where would the cheer and goodwill that are part of hospitality have come from? Janelle felt more hopeless than ever.

She went into a deep depression, crying throughout the day and waking up at night to cry too. She questioned her decision to stay with Mark and take care of him. If her counselor had let Steve and Joan off the hook so easily, maybe Janelle's decision to stay had been misguided. What did her sacrifice mean, if any-thing? She had believed so strongly she was doing the right thing, the loving thing, the moral thing. What if she had run away, taken the easy way out, like the Radleys had? Maybe she had been a chump. Maybe, and the thought made her cry again, she had wasted her life.

Perspective was slow in coming. Eventually she realized that Steve was grieving the loss of his brother, and hadn't been able to tell Mark how painful it was to lose him. "If only we had been able to talk, just sit down, all four of us, and say what we felt," Janelle grieved. "We could have told them how much we missed them, and they could have told us how much it hurt to see Mark get sicker. Maybe we could have worked out a compromise." She says now, "We both lost." She struggled to convince herself that Steve's actions weren't just the result of cowardice and selfish-ness, and at length she made peace with what had happened, accepting it as one more casualty of Mark's illness. She says, "As hard as those times were, at least I was there when Mark was still Mark."

In her heart of hearts, Janelle realized that she stayed partly because she was Mark's wife. She'd promised him. Watching Mark get sicker had been so grinding for her, she understood why Steve had bolted. She'd been tempted herself.

It's human nature to avoid life's unpleasant realities—that reluctance is why no one likes to visit nursing homes. Those places, and their sad tenants, remind us of the fate that awaits all of us sooner or later. We who have partners there don't have the luxury of staying away.

Norma Imber says, "It's so funny, when someone dies at the nursing home, I look at the obit, and I see this person had five children, fourteen grandchildren. And I think, where were they? It's very common." She had her own problems with their five children—her three and Robert's two—after he went into the nursing home.

When she married him, her children were 14, 11, and 5, and his boys, 18 and 15. "We all got along wonderfully. It was like a party," she says. She believed her kids loved Robert as much as she did, but a year after his stroke, she found out differently. Visiting Robert in the nursing home, she called her youngest daughter, then handed the phone to Robert. After some pleasantries, he handed the phone back. "Don't you ever do that again," her daughter's voice said coldly. Norma was stunned. "Do what?" she asked. "You know what," said her daughter. That conversation was her first inkling that her children weren't going to rally around Robert. "When I asked them why, they said, in a kind way, it's your problem, not ours," she remembers. "It was a heartbreak, a terrible time."

She thinks her children began to withdraw when they realized Robert was not going to get better, but she has never been brave enough to confront them about it. Through prayer, journaling, and counseling with a rabbi at the nursing home, she decided to forgive them. "I came to the conclusion that, come holidays, I wasn't going to sit there by myself. I wanted to be with my children." On holidays, she visits Robert first, then goes to one of their homes. Their withdrawal still pains her, especially when she sees families visiting at the nursing home, but her children always include her in their celebrations, which has made it easier to allow them their distance from Robert.

Lack of support from children we believed were raised to be caring is a bitter disappointment. Bob Keller's voice grows heated when he talks about his stepdaughter's lack of concern for her mother, his wife, Ellen. Ellen took only six months "to go from viable to vegetable," as Bob describes her rapid descent into Alzheimer's dementia. He's furious that much of Ellen's earnings as a nurse went to put Katie through nursing school, which was "not a cheap deal," Bob says. Ellen had only a few months after diagnosis when she was still herself, but while Katie's husband's parents had a cabin across the lake from Bob and Ellen's, Katie never came to visit. Now that Ellen is in a nursing home, bed-bound, unable to recognize anyone, Bob can't forgive Katie. One day, unable to stifle his rage any longer, he called her and lectured her on repaying Ellen's sacrifice and love with greed and neglect. Knowing that Katie's husband was probably behind her actions, Bob chewed him out too. "I left her crying and him mad," he says with satisfaction. "I told him if you were in arm's reach, you'd be madder yet, 'cause I'd belt you into the middle of next month." Afterward, he felt relieved. "I simmered down considerably." Bob's son tells him, not entirely in jest, that he's going to be sure to attend Ellen's funeral just to keep Bob from causing a riot.

When life is going well, love abounds and harmony reigns. In the glow of good times, we believe the bonds of friendship will only get stronger. As soon as the hard times set in, some of the people we considered friends suddenly remember prior commitments. Cracks appear in what seemed like rock-solid alliances. Chronic illness separates true friends from the hangers-on. "Most of the time, the people you consider friends aren't friends at all," one wife said. "They're just people you know." Another husband takes the concept further. "True friends come over and toilet your wife when you're gone," he says. Norma Imber says that one couple has stood by her. The husband in this couple was her first husband's best man, and although Richard died suddenly over thirty years ago, "We continue to be friends through all of this," she marvels. She goes out with them every Tuesday, no matter what little disasters the day has brought. She hasn't been quite so lucky with others. "With one couple, the wife will call to see how everything is, and that's it. They do nothing more than that. And with another, the husband comes every Friday to visit my husband. That's it. Period."

Losing a friend hurts even in the best of circumstances, but when you're desperate for emotional support, the loss cuts deeply. Margo Brooke's husband, Monte, had ALS for five years. She understood that, faced with Monte's illness, friends felt helpless. "They kept asking, 'What can we do, what can we do?'" she says. "Not having things in common anymore was a problem too. What do you talk about?" Only a few friends stayed with her and their family through it all: one couple friend, one friend of his, and new friends of hers, a family. With rare insight, she says that the new friendship worked because "they could take us where we were, in the now, instead of bringing in the past. The relationship was going forward instead of looking backward. Other friends would compare where we were with where we had been and couldn't handle it."

As Janelle's story shows, we suffer for our mates, too, when friends fall away. One man, who takes care of his wife with MS at home, laments, "The beautiful, intelligent, talented, lively, energetic, socially active, charming, and sexy woman I married . . . has become a totally dependent, childlike person with huge physical and cognitive disabilities." But he feels that the final indignity for her is that, although she is still interested in other people, other people are not interested in her. He says, "Her former 'friends' cannot spare even two minutes a month to call her and say hello. She is lonely for female conversation, and try as I might, that is one skill I will never learn."

When we spend twenty-four hours a day, seven days a week with our spouses, we can't understand why their "friends" can't spare a few minutes for them. A woman whose son has gone into the same business as his MS-stricken father deals with some of the same people his dad did. She says, "When Jeff talks to these people, they'll say, 'Well, how's your dad?' And it just pisses Jeff off. He thinks, 'You live right here in town, why don't you call him?' One day Jeff was talking to one of these people and got the same old question. So Jeff said, 'Bob, you live a whole lot closer to him than I do, you could give him a call.' And Bob said, 'You're right, Jeff. I could.'"

Jill found it galling that after her husband Ralph's horse-riding accident, which left him brain-damaged and partially paralyzed, his friends in the Elks ignored him. Ralph had been a lifelong member, and a selfless worker for the group. "My husband was a professional volunteer," she says. "Anyone could call him, any day, any hour, he would go. He never said no. Never." After Ralph's accident, in spite of the inconvenience, Jill loaded him and his wheelchair into the car and took him to the church they had attended for years. She remembers, "Once in a while, an Elk would stop and say, 'How ya doing, Pal?' But mostly, people would walk right past us. They'd say, 'Good morning,' but they wouldn't ask if they could help me. They wouldn't even hold the door for us." She changed to a congregation that fewer of Ralph's friends attended, and didn't look back.

Through a friend, Jill heard about a nondenominational group of trained volunteers who visit shut-ins. She called a church that had the program and begged for someone to visit Ralph and talk about "man things," like fishing and hunting. At first the minister was reluctant because they weren't members of his congregation, but then said he'd make an exception in their case. Jill was dismayed when the volunteer turned out to be a woman. To Jill's surprise, however, she was very good with Ralph, and Jill found herself looking forward to the volunteer's visits, as regular as sunrise, and the two became friends. When she left after two years, a male volunteer, equally compassionate, took her place. Ralph's speech is difficult, but "this man has gotten so good at understanding him," Jill says.

"Friends feel very helpless when chronic illness hits," says Shevy Healey, a clinical psychologist who has worked extensively with the chronically ill and their spouses. "They're reminded of their own vulnerability, and they get scared. It's a brave person who will hang in there with a friend with chronic illness." She recommends sitting down and talking with friends who are withdrawing. "It may seem uncomfortable in the beginning, but simply say, 'We're the same people we always were, we're your friends, we'd like to see you, and if some things make you uncomfortable, let's talk about them.'" Healey admits this method doesn't guarantee results. "You need to reach out to old friends and take your chances, and reach out to new ones as well." She says that, often, new friends will be those with some experience with illness. "That's why support groups are so good."

Anger at old friends' leaving can blind us to new friends coming into our lives. Sometimes casual acquaintances draw closer and become friends indeed. These new friends who don't have a history with us are more likely to "take us where we are," as Margo Brooke discovered. I think of one man, a neighbor of ours, who never failed to visit once a week and read *Sports Illustrated* to Don at the nursing home, something I didn't like to do. Another couple we'd known only casually before, the husband a coworker of Don's, visited regularly, bringing him a bottle of his favorite brandy on holidays. People who lend a hand during difficult times earn a special place in our hearts. Sometimes I wished that all our friends could know how comforting their mere presence was. I knew they couldn't fix anything; if there were a fix, we would have done it ourselves long ago. Just by showing up, friends give us a unique gift, the gift of themselves. If they can listen without judging or giving advice, they're doubly appreciated.

I've written in an earlier chapter of callous doctors who add to our misery. Pat Oswald's husband was unfortunate enough to contract a rare neurological illness their local hospital hadn't encountered. Fifty-four-year-old Fran Oswald came home from his job as a photofinisher one evening in February complaining of feeling chilled. He and Pat had recently been sick with a bout of food poisoning, but Fran thought they had recovered. The next morning Fran tried to get up to go to the bathroom and fell out of bed, paralyzed from the knees down. Pat, horrified, called the paramedics, and he was rushed to the hospital. "Hour by hour his body stopped working. One hour he could hold his arm up, the next it was totally limp. It still haunts me terribly," she says. Dashing out for a quick dinner with her mother, she returned to find a nurse trying to stuff a croissant sandwich into Fran's mouth. By then, he had lost the ability to swallow. He turned to Pat, and in a strangled whisper, pleaded, "Help me. I'm dying." Pat ran for a doctor, who stopped the feeding, but had no idea what else to do. By the time Fran's Guillain-Barré syndrome was diagnosed several days later, he was quadriplegic.

Pat suspected that her husband's Guillain-Barré, a paralysis that can be brought on by a serious bacterial infection, came from eating take-out chicken. She had been violently ill from that meal too, but she recovered with no aftereffects. Fran wasn't so lucky. By the time his doctor began to administer plasmapheresis, a process that cleans the blood of toxins, Fran's neurological damage was irreversible. When the treatment failed to produce any improvement, the doctor asked Pat how long she and Fran had been married. "Twelve years," she replied. He laughed and said, "Well, at least you had twelve good years." With great presence of mind, Pat replied, "Fuck you. You're fired!" Fran lived another four years and two months as a quad. Is it any wonder, Pat says now, that "anger was my strongest emotion through this?"

Dorothea's husband has had a kidney transplant, but instead of being the magic bullet they thought would make him well, it only brought on a new set of problems. Ironically, the new kidney is healthy, but the medications he must take to keep from rejecting it have wreaked havoc on his body. Her husband recently went to the hospital when one of his legs became paralyzed from a blood clot, and while he was there, doctors found a blood clot in the other leg. Her fury is obvious when she says, "You go in with one thing and they go out of their way to find something you didn't know about." She believes, "Doctors don't cure anything. They just arrest things. They should be arrested, if you ask me."

Dorothea is like a punch-drunk fighter who never knows where the next blow will land. Like the rest of us, she only knows there's another blow coming. With so little known about the conditions our partners have—what caused them, what course they will take, how long they will last—our lives have been swallowed up by uncertainty. We look to the medical profession, which should be able to cure, and find that not only are doctors as helpless as we are, they can't even tell us what to expect. Jim Russell's wife, Hannah, has had MS for nine years. "The doctors have been no help whatsoever," he says. "She's been in hospitals all over the area, Yale–New Haven, Albert Einstein College of Medicine, St. Agnes, the MS clinic there, and to a bevy of other neurologists. We've seen them all. They don't even want to talk to the spouse. They're very cold." Maybe the coldness is defensiveness because they know they don't have any answers; whatever the reason, experiences like the Russells' are enough to make us swear off doctors forever.

So, like Pat Oswald, we fire the obnoxious ones and try to work with the good ones. Jim and Hannah Russell found one retired doctor who'd go out of his way for them. When they read about a black market drug that sounded promising, this doctor arranged to get some shipped from Bulgaria. The drug didn't have any effect, but they were grateful for his help. Often, family doctors who know us and our families take more of an interest than specialists who see us once.

No matter what the malady, doctors make handy targets, and get blamed unfairly for the fact that science doesn't know as much about certain diseases as others. In an age that replaces organs almost as easily as car parts, we have high, maybe unreasonable, expectations of the medical profession. Well spouses are among the most disillusioned medical consumers, because we know firsthand its limitations.

Anger, like a vicious dog, is difficult to control, and has a nasty way of biting us when our backs are turned. Its power is illustrated in this parable: You can keep the slaves chained in the cellar only so long. Then one dark night they rise up and burn down the house. We know that the last thing our partners want is to be sick, don't we? Yet we blame them for getting sick. Is this fair? No. Does it happen anyway? Oh yes, indeed it does.

When you hate your spouse for getting sick, you spin around and around in an endless cycle of anger, then shame because you feel angry, then anger because you feel ashamed. And finally you become furious that you're trapped and can't get out with any amount of self-talk. Margy and Joe Kleinerman had many plans for their retirement before Joe got Alzheimer's. Margy says, "We had planned to spend our golden years going on cruises and traveling, just in general enjoying each other. When I hear of a couple going on various trips to various places, I don't begrudge them their good fortune at all. They worked hard and they deserve it. But, gee, we worked hard too. You know, I want them to have everything, but I want me to have it too." Well-intentioned friends tell her that "life isn't fair," or "he can't help it, you know," but they're only lighting a short fuse. "I really get upset when people say things like that," says Margy. "Of course he can't help it. That has nothing to do with me being mad at him." She understands that her anger isn't touched by logic, and she's mad anyway. She directs it at her psychiatrist, who helps her deal with being mad at Joe. "I yell at her, that's what I pay her for," Margy says. "And the advantage of Joe's short-term memory loss is that he won't remember me yelling at him anyway."

In the alchemy of anger, denying it (psychologists call it "stuffing") only makes it more potent. Since Don's death, when I encounter someone who had a role in my "life with MS," I start by apologizing. "I hope I was nice to you," I say, "because I was so angry during those years." I remember yelling at a pharmacist for being out of a drug Don needed; criticizing the director of hospice for withdrawing care from my husband because he had stopped progressing enough to be a hospice patient anymore, "not dying fast enough," I termed it; yelling at another pharmacist for making a mistake on a bill; arguing with the director of the nursing home for charging exorbitantly for a speech therapist who wasn't helping Don at all. And I won't even start on the set-to's with home health aides who didn't show up or tried to take over our lives. No doubt I had cause to be angry. But I was too angry for the situation, and would have had better results with a gentler approach.

When we're constantly angry, we overreact. Dorothea wrote a letter to her husband's brother and his wife several years ago that cut off any further communication from them. She insists, "In regard to anger, the words that are yelled and the letters that are written are actually justified, I think. They're just not the wisest courses of action that could have been taken. But when one is in a true state of high piss, one doesn't consider anything but the moment, wisdom be damned." The problem is that once spoken, words can't be recalled. And they alienate the people we need most.

What well spouses are really furious at is the cosmic turn of events that brought us here, but how can we rage at that? So we find something nearer to hand, the doctor who delivers the news, the friends and family who abandon us, our unlucky spouses. Illness forces us to give up so much personal power, and feeling helpless and out of control is infuriating. One wife describes these increasing concessions as "being forced into progressively smaller boxes." When the people to whom we entrust control let us down, we're filled with rage. Some of us turn our anger on God, and find him a good outlet. As Linda Anderson says, "God doesn't say, 'You're mad, so you're out of the will.' God isn't threatened by my tears and my anger."

Our husbands and wives have their own anger to deal with; lashing out at them can be like pouring gasoline on a fire. If they don't fight back it feels worse. One wife wrote to *Mainstay* that she got angry with her husband because he wouldn't talk to her. "I got so mad that I lost control and hit him and pulled his hair. Ever since then, I have been living with enormous guilt." Her lack of control shocked her, but her husband's words heaped hot coals on her head: "He said he deserved it because he was sick." Don was not an angry MS-er, and for that, I can only thank God and fate. I was usually the one who flew off the handle, and he'd watch me stomp around and yell and slam cabinets until I had it out of my system. "I'm not mad at you. I'm mad at this disease," I'd say. He gave me the benefit of the doubt. "You have every right to be mad," he'd say. His mild answer usually had the effect of quenching the flames. When we got mad at each other, the disagreements most often arose over how to perform caregiving tasks. I'll discuss those later in this chapter.

For Bette Allbright, one of the first signs of her husband Jim's MS was an anger-control problem. Luckily, Bette recognized that his illness was behind the change and didn't return fire. Jim, who had been, in Bette's words, "the perfect father," became grouchy and intolerant. "Our children were real small at the time, and all of a sudden he had no patience. If they played, he would be yelling, 'Be quiet! Shut up! I can't take the noise.'" Jim also became forgetful, and that helped Bette put the puzzle pieces together.

Knowing that your partner's anger is the result of organic brain changes may help you control your own anger. Unfortunately, no medical tests at present can pinpoint whether the anger-control area in the brain has been compromised. A well spouse has to trust her instincts here, but if a husband or wife has begun to act angry in situations that didn't upset them in the past, and is also showing other behavior changes, maybe the anger is due to the illness. As the "normal" one in the relationship, you may feel even guiltier if you respond in kind to your partner's abuse, because you're "supposed" to be the strong one. For some reason, anger seeks its own level, and we can easily become as hostile as our partners if we don't deal with it constructively.

John Hardin's wife, Nancy, was twenty-nine when she developed a rheumatological illness doctors could not diagnose. It wasn't lupus, but it had many of the same symptoms, the worst of which was irritability. Like Bette Allbright's husband, Nancy found the normal commotion of their three growing children excruciating. In constant pain from her pelvis and lower back, she was always yelling at the kids to be quiet. Seven years into the illness, she began having seizures so severe she had to be hospitalized. The Nancy that came home after twelve days was a different woman.

The anoxia from the seizures had caused some brain damage, but had also mysteriously eliminated her pain. Although her speech was garbled, her temperament had mellowed dramatically, and the kids found her much easier to get along with. The downside to the change was that she had suffered some short-term memory loss, which made her so anxious she was afraid to let John out of her sight. "I couldn't get away from her," he says tiredly. "When you can't remember, you keep asking questions. And questions aren't bad, but when they become the same questions and the same routine, it starts to get annoying. And then there's no break from it, it's all day, all night, every day." John's patience wore thin. Gradually, as a result of a series of small strokes medication couldn't control, Nancy's temper assumed frightening proportions. In the "before" years, John could fire back. Now responding in kind could start an all-out war, with Nancy coming at him screaming, fists flailing. Her rage made her strong, and she would grab his beard with both hands and not let go. These episodes occurred once a week, and lasted at least an hour. During the lulls, John tried mightily to control his own temper, but sometimes, exasperated, he snapped at her, and the battle was on. Most of the time, however, "it just came out of nowhere, like somebody had flipped a switch," he says. When something set Nancy off, all John could do was wait for it to pass.

He thought about a nursing home, but he loved her and wanted to keep her at home. She could still dress herself, liked doing housework, and was still interested in sex. She had maintained her sense of humor, one of the things he loved most about her. "As she's gotten worse, it's become more childlike," he says, "but it's still her unique sense of humor." What keeps them together, more than anything, he says, is that "she still knows that she really loves me and wants to be with me."

Nevertheless, he wondered if keeping her home was wise. One beautiful summer night she became so psychotic she called the police, believing John was her first husband and was beating her. After they came and took her off to the psychiatric ward, John sat on the steps of their house, looking up at the stars and wondering if Nancy was out of his life forever. He remembered other episodes. One of her outbursts occurred when a friend who happened to have a master's in counseling was staying with them, and she suggested that John simply leave the house when Nancy got irate. Next time, John did exactly that. "I'd just put my shoes on, or get dressed quickly, and take off faster than Nancy could keep up with me." Sometimes that meant he was shirtless, but the method worked. "I'd just walk down the road, faster than she could keep up, and that was enough time." He'd always loved gardening, and sometimes in nice weather he would slip back to the house, sit down in the garden, and begin pulling weeds. "That's been very therapeutic on more than one occasion," he says, "getting in touch with something other than my anger."

Another of John's friends, whose mother was alcoholic when she was growing up, understood that Nancy's unpredictability was similar to someone on a drinking binge, and offered a sympathetic ear. After the night the police came, Nancy spent a month in the psychiatric ward, where they gave her Haldol, a powerful antipsychotic drug that eliminated her temper tantrums. Putting Nancy in a day care center for Alzheimer's patients several days a week helped too, because she came home too tired to ask questions.

Unfortunately, although Nancy's anger has abated, John's anger continues to surprise and humiliate him. He is committed to keeping Nancy home, but the Haldol makes her urinate frequently, and if he isn't there to stop her, she goes anywhere. One night, when she tried to urinate standing up, he screamed at her. Even though Nancy doesn't remember his words, he is filled with remorse. "Anger is what I feel the stupidest and guiltiest about," he says.

Learning how to deal with anger, his and hers, has been an ongoing challenge for Kas and Ken Enger. They had been married for thirteen years when Ken got MS, and began to have problems controlling his temper. "He would just start having these outbursts," says Kas, "and no one knew when they were going to come, or why, or how. He had never done that when he was healthy." At first, Kas suffered in silence. She came from a family that "preferred martyr complexes to expressing anger," so she would keep to herself rather than talking about it with Ken. Then she made a discovery. One day when he started to yell, she yelled back. He immediately backed off and apologized. "It was kind of like a bucket of cold water in his face. It would kind of wake him up, and he'd go, Oh, OK. I thought, gee, I wish I'd done this years ago," she says.

She also learned to draw the line. One day they and their youngest daughter were getting ready to go somewhere, and Ken and Emily were waiting for Kas in the van. Ken, at the wheel, took offense at something Emily said, and reached around and grabbed her jacket to pull her toward him. He was still yelling at her when Kas got to the van and calmed them both down. Emily complained later to Kas, "Dad hit me." Kas told her she thought he had hit her by accident while reaching around to grab her jacket, but a few days later, she asked Ken if he had meant to hit Emily. He hadn't meant to, he told Kas. "Well, that's good," said Kas. "Because if you ever start hitting anybody in this family, I'm out of here. I will not tolerate that." She knows that Ken is not by nature a violent man, and that "as long as he's in control" he would not hit anyone. Kas realizes that dealing with Ken's anger has taught her to express her own. She doesn't lash out at him anymore as she did at first. "I know I still have a ways to go, but I'm more prone to tell him right away, instead of stuffing it and letting it grow until it blows."

According to Kas, one of their ongoing disagreements centers on caregiving. "Maybe it's just in my head, and maybe it's just coincidental," she confides. "But if I suggest something, whether it's let's move your leg over here, or let's try this exercise, or whatever, it seems like he's real determined, passively aggressively determined, that it's not gonna happen." His balkiness presents a problem when he falls. She says, "He always wants to do it his way. I'll look at him down on the floor, and say, 'OK, Emily, you get on one side and I'll get on the other, and we'll put our arms under his armpits and we'll just hoist him.' But he doesn't want to do that. He wants to roll over, he wants to get up on all fours, he wants to help by using his arms. Well, if he uses his arms, that leaves us nothing to pick him up with. That makes it really difficult, so usually we just kind of grab his pants and help hoist him, or whatever. But we just stand there and wait for him to tell us how he wants it done, and that's how we do it." Of course, such skirmishes are dwarfed by the size of the war, and Kas knows it. "Every time you think you've got a system down, things change, and then you have to change the system."

Anger is a special problem for women, because, as Kas noted, girls are socialized to be martyrs rather than fighters. Wives of sick men find themselves doing all the duties men perform without being allowed to vent like men. We mow the lawn, fix the faucets, do the taxes, but when we'd like to swear or put a fist through a window, we stop short. We pretend we're not hurt, and hope that the feeling will dissipate. Instead, it burns and builds until it blows. Women in our society are allowed to cry, not rage, and as a result, we're afraid of anger. As Kas found, women who are able to step out of the stereotype and express anger are more at peace than those who can't.

Maybe because our partners have so little control in the rest of their lives, they're doubly determined to control the things they can. Don hated feeling conspicuous, and even though I had our pastor's permission to pull onto the lawn to get closer to the front doors of the church, Don didn't want me to. I resented the fact that he couldn't sacrifice some vanity so that I wouldn't have to push him as far. Sometimes I parked on the grass over his objections; often I just gave in and parked in the parking lot.

Waiting on a spouse hand and foot is difficult even if they're appreciative and don't take advantage, but when they're manipulative and demanding, hostile and hard to please, a saint's halo would slip. Even the gentlest caregiver gives in to anger on occasion. Bill Hill, whose wife, Peggy, an Alzheimer's patient, has a hospital bed in their living room, claims, "It's a privilege to take care of her." Yet he admits that he "hit her once on the butt" because she was fighting him during a diaper change. He was stunned. "I can't describe my feelings after I did that," he says. "I had never touched her like that before." They had always been "kissy-kissy" when Peggy was well.

Illness changes the dynamics of marriage, so that a system that worked when both were healthy can become ruinous. Roy Layton describes himself this way: "I guess I've been a giver all my life. I have a serious tendency to just dedicate myself to other people." So it was natural that in their marriage, his wife, Donna, was "the director," and he was the "worker." "Let's put a shelf here, Honey," she would say, and Roy would happily oblige, while Donna fetched and carried. They made an efficient team, to his mind. When she became ill, she couldn't help him anymore, but she wasn't willing to relinquish her director role. Quite the opposite; she became more and more demanding, while Roy got angrier and angrier. One incident stands out. He had just set her on the toilet, and gone into another room, when she called him with another little request. He asked her if there was anything else he could do while he was there, and she said no. He headed back to the family room and had no sooner gotten seated in the recliner when she called him again. She wanted him to "straighten up her perfume bottle on the mirror tray," or something "of that degree of validity," he says. Roy saw red. "I picked up her wheelchair and threw it against the door," he says, "and the little wheely bar stabbed into the back of the door, so that the wheelchair remained suspended above the floor." He says sadly, "A wheelchair is kind of an awkward thing to throw." But at least it hadn't been Donna. He never abused his wife physically, he says, although he admits he was verbally abusive on occasion. Demoralized by her trivial demands, he eventually divorced her. "I was at the bottom," he says. "I was thoroughly convinced that her MS would kill me before it killed her."

Physical abuse does occur in these marriages, however, although no one knows how often. One woman wrote to the newsletter *Mainstay* that she had scars on her ankles from her husband's using his wheelchair as a weapon.

Anger, when there's so much of it, slops over onto everyone, and trying to decipher, in the heat of the moment, whether or not it's directed at us can be difficult. Mark Johannes says of his wife, Bonnie, "Right now, my biggest problem is putting up with the tempers, the tantrums Bonnie has over her own body, that it doesn't work. She gets very angry. One time we were getting ready for bed. I was sitting on the bed, and she was trying to transfer into bed. And remember, I don't even get half the bed anymore, I only get a third. So here I am sitting on the bed, and I hear this 'Move, you son of a bitch!' Here she is, throwing the mule skinner blues out in my direction, but not at me. She was talking to her legs. She was trying to move. She can hardly drag one foot even a couple of inches anymore. Once I realized it wasn't directed at me, it was better."

As I said in Chapter 2, husbands and wives can clash on the question of who owns the illness, and disagree endlessly on the proper things to eat, what medications to take, what treatments to try, or whether to try anything at all. Each of us comes to marriage with beliefs about our own effectiveness in the world that were probably in place by the time we were four years old. These are fundamental to our personalities, determining such things as whether we vote Republican or Democrat, whether we go to church on Sunday, even whether we're willing to circulate a petition in the supermarket. Naturally, beliefs that are so central to our identities can be hard to change. If your partner is a "can-do" type who wants to travel to distant places in search of a cure, and try everything he reads about, but you're less sanguine about whether a cure for the illness exists anywhere, conflict will arise. If you're convinced your partner is simply rolling over, you're the one that's going to be frustrated at his or her inaction. Chuck and Polly never resolved their disagreement about Polly's eating habits, and Chuck couldn't help taking her refusal to curb her calories personally. He needed a year of counseling to get over his anger at her. "She never stopped looking for the magic bullet," he says. Linda Anderson says, "I would get angry at Steve for not trying. He was a gentle man, and didn't have much of what I call 'the fighting spirit.' Sometimes I felt him giving up, and I'd think, 'This doesn't have to overtake you emotionally too.'"

As our partners disintegrate, we may switch roles. Pat Oswald looked at Fran's wasted body and couldn't understand why he wanted to live. Yet Fran insisted on a feeding tube and full life support. After three years passed with no change in his condition, Pat wanted him to stop. "It's not that I wanted him to die," she explains. "I just thought, 'My God, he doesn't know when to quit.' I couldn't help being mad." Sometimes she'd suggest that it was time "to give up the ship," but the angry glare she got was the proverbial look that could kill. Many times she stormed out, only to find that by the time she reached home she was awash in guilt. "I was afraid he'd think I didn't want him to live." She reflects, "I learned, through this experience, that there are fates worse than death."

Others spoke of partners who insist on being resuscitated time and again (one wife said her husband had been revived seven times), or given massive amounts of antibiotics when infection sets in, only to be delivered back into the world of endless dying. If the patient is lucid enough to make his wishes known, doctors must honor those, not the spouse's, although our lives hang in the balance too. In the last year of Don's life, when he wanted antibiotics for infections that would have carried him off peacefully, and I objected, he quoted Dylan Thomas to me: "Do not go gentle into that good night, Chrissie." After his death, I had several dreams in which he was alive again, and in the same ravaged condition. Nightmares.

All emotions serve an evolutionary purpose, and anger is no exception. Anger tells us something. Usually it says that our boundaries have been breached, that someone is intruding on our territory. With our territory already feeling so constricted, no wonder we're mad all the time. Anger is a servant, bringing messages about our well-being. And in order to keep it from burning down the house, it must be acknowledged and dealt with. Not to do so is to court disaster.

The methods we choose can help us or hurt us. While tempting, turning to alcohol is no more of an escape for well spouses than for anyone else. Jim Russell knows. "After Hannah's diagnosis, I started to drink a lot. I was angry at the situation. I think a lot of well spouses turn to alcohol for an escape," he says. As he realized, alcohol is a depressant, and God knows we don't need that. He got into an AA program and has been sober ever since. Many well spouses take antidepressants, and these can be helpful in improving one's mood. These drugs can provide the boost a spouse may need to make positive changes in his or her life, and to begin to create a life separate from the illness.

If most of our anger is the result of feeling cheated, the antidote is to feel less cheated. But first, recognize that your anger is completely justified. You and your spouse got a bad deal. If you're always telling yourself you shouldn't feel an emotion that is justifiable, you're going to be even angrier. While uncomfortable, your anger is natural and healthy and entirely appropriate.

If anger is energy, how can well spouses best direct it so that it works for them, rather than against them? The spouses who were coping best acknowledged that they couldn't change the course of the illness or how their partners dealt with it and that those things were simply out of their control. The only things they could change were themselves. With surprising perception, one told me, "I've realized that the angrier I am at my husband, the less I've taken responsibility for myself." So the next question is, What do you need to make your situation bearable?

Denise, whose husband has kidney disease and whose son was an alcoholic, says, "I joined a program to help me rack my brain on doing everything I could to help my son, and ended up realizing I could only change myself." She applies this philosophy to her husband's twelve-year illness. "I'm powerless over his disease, and powerless over his behavior. I have to let it go." Others learned in counseling to "accept the things they couldn't change," and found that, paradoxically, letting go was empowering, because it freed energy that could be used in more constructive ways. Denise has applied that acceptance to her husband's hostility and emotional abuse, which she attributes to his illness. Instead of arguing with him, she swims four times a week, takes yoga, and goes to the gym. She is committed to staying with him, and these activities keep her sane.

Each of us has to identify what well spouse Eugenia Staerker calls the "pockets of pleasure" in each day. You can't be either a good caregiver, if that is your aim, or a happy person without devoting time and attention to your own needs. Remember, one life to a customer. Find out what renews you, even if it's only for a little while. Exercise was the number one choice for getting rid of anger among those I interviewed. Well spouses also mentioned journaling, praying, playing musical instruments, chatting online to others who either did or didn't know that they were well spouses (depending on their needs), doing yoga, participating in support groups, spending time with children—the list is as various as the people it comprises.

How can you find the time? You have to ask for it—a big hurdle, maybe the biggest of all, for many of us. We've been taught from the cradle that self-sufficiency is the great American virtue, and being a well spouse means having to unlearn, or at least modify, that lesson—or become miserably isolated. Is it fair that you have to spell out your needs to friends and relatives who should be more perceptive? No. But we must get past the injustice of having to ask and do it anyway. We must begin to see asking for help as a strength, not as a weakness.

Well spouses often forget that they have a right to their own decisions. When Don began to get frequent infections and I was getting whiplash racing to the nursing home, I took it up with a counselor. "He can't have it both ways," she told me. "He has to decide if he's going to live or die. If he's going to get antibiotics, it means that you don't have to rush up there every time he gets an infection. If he's going to die, you may want to be there."

Making spouses accountable leads to another avenue of help—our spouses. Illness skews the power base in a marriage so that our partners seem to have all the rights, and we have none. We slip into thinking that, because they're sick, their lives are the only ones that matter, and society encourages this belief. That thinking is appropriate in crisis situations, but taking a crisis mentality into a long-term situation doesn't work. We come to believe that their battle is the only real one, that their needs are the only ones that count. But this thinking isn't just unfair to us; it's unfair to them too. When we ask them to give what they still can, they are empowered. Can he go to bed when you do, so that you don't have to get up in the middle of the night to put him to bed? Can she wish you godspeed as you disappear for a weekend? Having the blessings of our spouses can be the nudge we need to enjoy ourselves away from them. Just because they're sick doesn't mean they don't have gifts to give. Expecting our partners to be givers as well as takers reminds them they are still in the family system, and that we expect them, as much as they are able, to act like partners.

Don once told me, "You don't have to catch every fly ball that's hit to you. You can let a few go by." That message applies to all of us. Unthinking health professionals assume that just because we're the spouses, we're the slaves. It's perfectly acceptable to say no sometimes—whether the task is diapering, catheterizing, toothbrushing, disimpacting. If we simply can't tolerate doing something, someone else can be found who doesn't mind doing those things. In the heat of the moment, we may forget we have choices, but we always do.

Dealing with anger on a strictly physical level is helpful too. Over the years I've learned never to throw out a light bulb. When thrown against a basement or garage wall, they have a wonderful loud crash that always makes me feel better. Someone mentioned putting a melon in a pillowcase and swinging it against a tree. I've parked the car in a deserted spot and screamed and pounded on the steering wheel for twenty minutes.

Well spouses are often sleep-deprived, and fatigue intensifies every emotion. Consider hiring someone to care for your spouse a couple of nights a week so you can sleep, or take an afternoon nap. The restorative power of sleep makes the whole world look brighter.

Keeping a journal is an excellent way to relieve stress. I have poured out every manner of emotion to my journal, which is never too tired or involved in its own life to listen. And it's free. I can spew poison onto the pages in the form of letters that will never be sent. I can talk to people who are dead, and rewrite situations so that they have happy outcomes. I can record my dreams and set goals. When I'm angry at someone, getting the words onto the page is cathartic, and when I close the book, I feel as if I've put away those feelings in a safe place. A journal can be a place to list, each day, one thing to be grateful for, something all well spouses need to keep in mind. It's also a place to record funny incidents and jokes to look back at when you need a smile. Another benefit of journaling: Reading about past crises you coped with reassures you that you can deal with the next one. For well spouses, this aspect alone can be very comforting. When we journal, we write the history of our lives, creating an anchor to hang on to when the storms howl. Some books to help you get started are listed in the bibliography.

Pat Oswald had been in therapy before Fran's illness, and

remembered how effective batakas, big soft bats to beat on pillows, were in getting rid of anger. With her two cats and two dogs in the house, however, she was afraid using batakas would terrorize them, so she bought some baseball bats and beat on a brick dog run outside her house. "I broke three baseball bats in six months," she says. "It helped."

The value of friends and family—a good support system—can hardly be overstated. Many of those I spoke to said they couldn't survive without support groups. Surprisingly, there's often a lot of laughter at these—black humor, to be sure, but especially comforting for its irreverence. Laughter is one of the best ways of cutting life's miseries down to size. "Friendship doubles our joys and divides our sorrows" are words for well spouses to live by. Talking about your frustrations with other well spouses is a great release. Support group members speak of the relief of knowing others are going through the same things, and that murderous thoughts are perfectly understandable when you've been awakened for the third time to fix a leaky catheter or stretch a cramping muscle. The Well Spouse Foundation, listed in the back of this book, keeps a list of support groups in various towns.

Friends may not have "answers" for us, because there aren't any answers, but they allow us to laugh and cry and feel less alone, and that makes a heavy burden a little lighter. "Sometimes the only sense you can make out of life is a sense of humor," read a card someone sent me.

Finding a friend who is willing to listen and won't try to fix you or your life is a tremendous help in letting off steam. I wore out a friend this way, however, and found I was more comfortable paying a counselor than risking my friendships. As Margy Kleinerman says, "That's what I pay my shrink for."

By treating ourselves with as much kindness as we treat our spouses, and finding a way to live fully in spite of this experience, we—and this is the ultimate goal for anyone who feels cheated by life—arrive at an attitude of forgiveness. We learn to say, I got a dirty deal, and so did my husband or wife. When we feel less depleted, because we're attending to our own needs, we begin to forgive life for the injustice it did us. We find we're not as angry as often.

# 7. Parenting: Raising Good Kids in Spite of the Illness

 Unlike in a divorce, the question of who gets the kids when chronic illness hits is a foregone conclusion: the well parent. In addition to our other duties, well spouses feel we must somehow be not just good-enough parents, like everyone else, but extra-good parents, to compensate for the deprivations of having the other parent sick. As one man said, "When Marie got MS, everyone in the family got MS."

Dr. Spock called children "our visible immortality." No one would deny that raising children is the most important job we do, but when our partners have a chronic illness, it falls a notch in the hierarchy. Rather than being parented, our children can end up doing the parenting—sometimes from a young age. They learn early that their needs come second, maybe third or fourth. They lose the option of saying no to the sick parent's requests, and feel guilty for resenting him or her. They aren't allowed temper tantrums because it might upset the emotional equilibrium in the household. They must be quieter, and cleaner, and more patient than other children. They feel guilty for resenting the fact that the family revolves around the sick parent. They worry excessively about the sick parent dying—and the well parent too. They worry about the well parent succumbing to the demands of the sick one. They feel freakish because, unlike their friends, their dad or mom is in a wheelchair. Denied a normal childhood, they become hyper-responsible and world-weary before their time

What to tell my children about Don's diagnosis was the first big question I faced. Megan and Tim were little when Don started having trouble walking—Tim was eighteen months, and Meg was four. Yet even though I had no answers myself, I knew I had to provide some for my children. The words were not as important as making the attempt. Over the months, I had tried not to cry in front of them, but they would have noticed my worried silences, and that their daddy wasn't walking right. They would have sensed a change in the emotional atmosphere the way small animals sense changes in the burrow. I knew that my son would have a very different childhood than his sister, who had been raised till now by two healthy parents. He would never know the luxury of having the family's attention shine only on him and his accomplishments. Instead, the focus would have to be on Don and his needs. I felt so sad for him.

I knew enough child psychology to know that little children indulge in magical thinking, so in their worlds, they are all-powerful. If they had ever felt angry at Don, and wished he would die, they would see his illness as something they had caused and feel guilty for making their dad sick. I knew also that I had to open the dialogue, that this was only the first of many talks we would have, that the children needed to feel they could ask about their dad, that we had to be able to put words to this unwelcome reality. From the beginning, I wanted them to see MS as our common enemy. It might take a lot of things away from us, but it couldn't take the love we had for each other. Talking about it seemed the logical first step in convincing them that having something bad happen to us didn't make us bad people—a message I knew they would have to hear again and again.

One night I set down the book I was reading to them. It was Meg's favorite, about thirteen bears, each of whom designs its own home. "Dad has a disease that makes his legs weak," I began. "His legs get tired real easily, like when you've been running for a long time. That's how it feels to him." I watched their faces as they took this in. Tim had fallen off a slide a week earlier, and the left side of his face looked like someone had smeared it with raspberry jam. I had watched him—from too far away, I realized too late—as his small form, curly blond head bobbing, climbed the steps of the slide, then missed the last step. As he began his tumble, I sprinted breathlessly toward him, knowing the effort was futile, that I would never arrive in time to break his fall. I could only clutch him to me, soothe his cries, wipe the blood away. I felt like that now. "Is Dad going to die?" Megan asked. I was relieved she could ask the question, but was momentarily stumped. I hadn't expected this question so soon. I tried to be honest but reassuring. "People with Dad's disease usually live as long as everyone else. Dad isn't going to die any time soon." I gathered them to me, one in each arm. "You didn't make Dad get this disease," I said. "Even if you got mad at him and wished he would die, it didn't make him get this, you know?" Their faces looked thoughtful. I picked up the book again, and we fled into the world of ursine architecture.

What had we done? I worried when it became clear that Don had a disease with a genetic component. It wasn't bad enough that my children were about to have their childhoods stolen. They also had to grow up with the specter that they might develop MS themselves someday. Still, I was selfishly glad they had been born before Don got MS, for not having them, their beauty, their robust health, their funny sayings and doings, was unthinkable. In those dark days when we first realized Don had something serious, the kids were my sanity. Changing diapers and cooking meals and reading storybooks kept my hands and vision · steady. The children were a noisy, tangible reminder of a world without MS.

We tried to keep things as normal as possible for them. We would deal with things one step at a time, I reminded myself, with the kids' needs as with everything else. Illness is humbling in the way it shoves you down and says, "Now, I'm in charge." I was grateful that at least we would have time to adjust gradually.

Children of chronic illness grow up fast. Don Crawford says of his daughter, Abbi: "She was full-grown at six. She had to be." Seeing a parent wither robs childhood of its innocence. Our children will never harbor the delusion that bad things happen only to other people. Yet, even as we grieve for them, we realize this awareness has its advantages. For one thing, they see every day how families take care of each other, and how their efforts make a difference. I'm sure they resented hearing me say this—and if I said it once, I said it a hundred times—"You're not the only one in this family. There are four of us here, and we have to do what's best for everybody."

I fretted about all that my children were missing, forgetting that maybe they were gaining something too. I was surprised to hear my daughter's third-grade teacher praise her resilience. "So many kids are afraid to try anything because they might fail. Not Megan," she enthused. I explained our home situation. "That's it, then," she said as she nodded. "Don't you think that if someone's had something major go wrong in their lives, the little things don't bother them? I think that's the way it is with her." I left the conference with my first glimmer that maybe my children's growing up wouldn't be an unrelieved disaster.

And our kids do turn out all right, even better than all right. Many children with chronically ill parents choose the medical field or other helping professions, becoming doctors and nurses and social workers and psychologists and teachers. In my interviews, these were the words well spouses often used to describe their children: "caring," "tender-hearted," "compassionate," "sensitive."

But mostly they were talking about adult children, not angry grade-schoolers or rebellious adolescents. Kids are angry, and rightly so, about the steady theft of a mother's or father's abilities. They dislike feeling different from their peers, and having a dad or mom in a wheelchair is the equivalent of wearing a brand. The day my eight-year-old son came home from school with a split lip and a black eye, I was mystified. I knew him to be an affable, cooperative third-grader. "This boy said my dad couldn't do anything," he told me, his eyes spilling over. I understood how painful it was for him to have a dad who was different.

Anger is the prevailing emotion in many homes, and while some spouses may permit their partners' directing it toward them, they draw the line when it comes to the kids—and they should. Steve Kambich made the nursing-home decision partly because the personality changes his wife, Wendy, suffered made her too angry at their children. "They were trying to be normal little kids, and if they spilled a little milk or something, she'd yell at them, and that just wasn't her," Steve says. One hair-raising day he came home to find his four-year-old daughter leaning over a stove with all the burners blazing. She was wearing only a nylon nightshirt. His wife had gone to the basement to do laundry, but couldn't crawl back upstairs. She was so determined to lead a normal life in spite of her MS that she wasn't using good judgment anymore. Steve decided then and there that Wendy needed a nursing home.

"I'm pretty protective of my boys," says Diane Maxwell. She would be the first to admit that she hasn't been able to protect her sons against all aspects of Jim's illness. "Jim was diagnosed in 1976, and Tyler, our second son, was born in 1980," she says. "Jim had been in remission for three years, so we thought everything was going to be great. Even though we had talked to Corey and Tyler about MS, it wasn't real to them in any way." Unfortunately, Jim's first bad exacerbation caused big problems for the little boys. "Corey said 'Monster,' and had nightmares, because Jim's eye drooped, and he was drooling and staggering, and his face was twitching." Diane says, "I tried to validate their feelings. I said, 'Remember how chemotherapy took Grandma's hair away? But inside she was still the person who loved you.' " Interestingly, she found that helping them process their fears helped her get perspective on these changes too.

Jim's facial symptoms didn't last. On the other hand, his impatience and verbal abuse have been an enduring problem. Diane's conflict about the situation is obvious when she says, "When I find myself or the boys tiptoeing around him, and I say, 'Don't tell Dad, 'cause it'll upset him' and 'Let's keep this a secret,' I know how dysfunctional that is." But the alternative is subjecting herself and her sons, now teenagers, to Jim's carping. She says that things are better than they were, and she doesn't have to be as watchful, largely because she helped the boys empower themselves. "They saw a counselor, somebody really good with children," she says. "She worked with them on mentally finding a space when they were confused or upset, and they could go to their space. She'd have them draw a mental circle around themselves, like a cocoon, and find that space, and think about what was real, and what they could change, and all those things. That has really helped them."

The counselor also helped them find a code word when Jim launched into a tirade at one of them. "Corey will walk by me and say, 'Duck's back,' and that means just let it roll off you like water off a duck's back," Diane says. "And I tell them, remember that that's just Dad, with a mixture of MS and medicine, and Dad loves you and would not say those things to hurt you in a million years." The arrangement has become something they do for each other. "They remind me of it and occasionally I remind them of it." Hearing Jim peck at her children has been one of the most painful side effects of his illness. "Sometimes, I'll say, 'Corey, or Tyler, I'm so sorry,' and they'll say, 'It's OK, Mom, just remember Duck's back.' And they'll lift me."

She is wise enough to recognize that their house doesn't have to be a battle zone. "We can't just be dealing with every crisis as it happens, every hour," she says. "We have to have strategies to get through it, so that we come out somewhat whole at the end of the day, or the week, or the month. And still have ourselves and some kind of vision for our own lives." And sometimes Jim can be a supportive parent. Diane makes a special effort to get him to the boys' bowling tournaments and football games. Jim "saves up" for these events by sleeping most of the previous day, and is exhausted afterward, but these family outings are rewarding for all of them.

Jonathan Ivey's wife, Louise, has been operated on three times for a recurring brain tumor, and as a result has memory and judgment deficits. The most disturbing thing to him is that his two daughters, now eight and twelve, have learned to tune their mother out. Their disobedience bothers him because, he says, "What Louise could be, as far as mothering, and what the kids allow her to be, are two different things. The problem is, she'll try to get the kids to do something they really should be doing, and I'll have to back her up. And other times, it's really not an appropriate activity for the kids, and I'll have to go against her. It's an ongoing issue, what best to do."

The whole family is currently in counseling, but Jon isn't sure if the situation can improve. A nagging question is whether the girls' disobedience is a reaction to his wife's inappropriate demands, or whether it's simply because of their growing independence. Besides the constant strain of being a referee, Jon worries about the level of hostility in the household. "Louise is an angry person," he says, adding that he doesn't know if her anger is a result of her brain surgeries or because of her frustration at her own limitations. He consoles himself that he, at least, has a good relationship with the girls, and sometimes he catches glimpses of their old life. "There have been good times for the four of us, like when we go to the zoo, or on picnics. It's not the same as it used to be, but it can still be good on some level."

Another man, whose wife is seriously brain damaged, faces a similar challenge. He is distressed that his sons, ages seven and nine, are starting to ignore his wife. He understands that this is happening because she cannot respond to them, but he has developed some rituals he hopes will help. Every night he reads the three of them a bedtime story, and at every opportunity, he reminisces about what his wife was like before the accident. He knows he can't force his sons to have a relationship with her, but can only provide an example by his own actions.

Jake, whose wife has had diabetes for twenty-five years, recalls how her illness affected their younger son, Doug. "When Doug came home from school, his mom would be in her chair, too tired to give him a glass of milk and a cookie like his friends' moms could do for them. Instead, she'd ask Doug to do things for her—

get her some water, close the window or door, get a blanket—small things to ask, but Doug resented it. He didn't have a mom there for him like his friends did. He refused to bring his friends home with him after school or invite them to stay overnight because 'his mom wasn't nice to them.'"

As in an alcoholic home, kids don't know what awaits them when they come in the door. Bringing friends into the situation is too risky. And they learn that once they enter the house, they can be asked to do any number of tasks they'd rather not do—emptying the trash and feeding the dog, as in other homes, or emptying a catheter bag or helping Mom onto the toilet, unlike in other homes. My daughter recalls feeling angry that, after Don went to the nursing home, she had to help me get him up from his nap when I brought him home on Sunday afternoons. I tried to have the kids take turns, because even with the Hoyer lift, getting Don out of bed was a two-person job. "I'd be having fun at someone's house, and then I had to drop it and come home," Megan says. "I hated that."

"There's so much more I have to expect from the kids than just the typical kid things," says Diane Maxwell. "They have to be there with their dad, walk with their dad, check on their dad. I've tried to instill in the kids that we're a partnership. We try to take turns doing things for Jim. If he needs a glass of water, one of us says, 'My turn.' Or one of us just does it. That's a reality we all have to accept, but I'm not going to make them do it, and not do it myself. It's my reality too."

Trying to spare kids from caregiving duties completely is as big a mistake as turning them into mini-slaves. Being involved in a parent's care, and being praised for it, teaches them the value of their own efforts, and gives them a sense of belonging. But as Diane Maxwell and Jon Ivey realize, the demands have to be balanced, whenever possible, by good times with the sick parent too.

As well partners, we have to facilitate this interaction. Don would get depressed that he couldn't be more involved in the kids' lives. "Why did God give me you and Timothy and Megan if I can't be a husband to you, and a father to them?" he'd say. I'd point out that even if he couldn't do physical things with them, he could still be a good father because he could listen. I told him that lots of able-bodied fathers are too busy to spend much time with their kids, so their able bodies don't help their kids much. Our culture puts so much emphasis on doing that we forget the greater importance of being—being with each other mindfully, and attending to each other's feelings and thoughts. In this way, he could be an excellent dad, and he was. As the kids were growing up, I tried to keep dinnertime a family time. After Don went to the nursing home, we had only Sunday dinners together, and I insisted that the kids, eleven and fourteen, keep that time free— not without a sulk sometimes. Over roast beef or chicken or Don's favorite, spaghetti, we read or recited poetry, played word games, told about one new thing we had learned the previous week, or just conversed. It was a time for airing grievances too. Those precious times held us together as Don slipped steadily from our lives.

Allowing kids time alone with us, so they can discuss the sick parent, is essential. For Diane Maxwell and her sons, the kitchen is their place to schmooze. "I have a real wide counter, and as babies they would sit in their little chairs. Now they stand in front of the counter." Currently, one son "is in a bake mood," and the other "likes salads," and cooking together "is a great time to connect with them," she says.

When Cathy Rammelsberg's husband developed kidney disease at age thirty-five, she spent long days with him at the hospital. But when four o'clock came, she drove home to her three daughters, the youngest of whom was a kindergartner. "We made dinner, spent the evening, and I put them to bed," she says. "People criticized me for not being at David's side night and day, but I needed to be home, so we had some normalcy to our lives." Carving out time for the kids proved worth the effort for Cathy, who says her daughters are very close to each other, and to her.

As our partners become sicker, it's easy to begin to exclude them from the life of the family, but doing this too soon is a disservice to them and our children. Even in his wheelchair, Don could help me discipline the kids. My mother, observing his technique, marveled at how quickly he could put out an arm and snag a child as neatly as netting a trout. Encircling one of them in his arms, he'd conduct an affectionate tête-à-tête, ending with, "That wasn't polite. Go tell your mother you're sorry."

Greta's husband, Curt, is quadriplegic with ALS, but she values his ability to set and enforce rules for their two teenage children, Sandy, age sixteen, and Brandon, age fourteen. "Curt is really good with the kids," she says. "He's pretty strict, we both are, and Sandy knows she can't cross the line with her father, while she will try to cross it with me. We stand as a front. I used to argue and fight with Sandy, but now I just tell her she needs to go and talk to her dad, and whatever he says, then I enforce it." Despite Curt's huge handicaps, Greta isn't ready to lose him yet. "I guess that's one of my real fears, that Curt will die before he can help Sandy and Brandon through this time."

The family wrangles over who will do things for Curt. "The kids just don't want to help him. Basically, Curt asks them to do very little, and I have to do more. Sometimes I get bitter about that," says Greta. She has tried to set rules for the children about their behavior when she has to leave them with Curt. "I've told them, if I'm not here and Dad's dependent on you, you cannot make him feel bad about needing your help."

She is grateful that somehow Brandon's best friend, Bobby,

who lives across the street and has been his friend "forever," isn't put off by Curt's condition. "When I have to send them to the basement so Curt can use the urinal, I just say, 'Now go downstairs for a while,' and they do, and that's just the way life is. Other friends might come and stay overnight now and then, but as far as having groups of friends hanging out on a regular basis, no."

"Did you feel like you lost touch with your children?" Greta asks plaintively. "I just feel like I have not been there for my children at all, for years now. I'm physically in the house all the time, but I'm always preoccupied with taking care of their dad." I told her that that was one of my biggest sadnesses about Don's illness, that because so much energy went into caring for him, not much was left over for the kids.

Decisions about how to spend my time caused me anguish. Don spent a week in the hospital in 1985 undergoing chemotherapy. Cyclophosphamide, a cancer drug, was being tried on MS as a way to kill off some of the white cells attacking the nervous system. Unfortunately, Don was too nauseated to last the entire seven days the treatment required, and signed himself out after only five. It was one of the lowest points in an ordeal that never lacked for low points. Both of us were exhausted and depressed. Desperate to get away, I made plans with a woman friend to go out to dinner in another town, then stay overnight and come home on Sunday. At 3:00 on Saturday afternoon, half an hour before we were to leave, Tim fell off his bike. He hadn't time to scramble up off the sidewalk when his friend, Russell, following closely behind, ran over his right ear, exposing a pearly wedge of cartilage. The accident, while unsettling, was minor, and the cut easily stitched closed. But now I wondered whether I should stay or go.

Tim was my less demanding child. Meg was the one who

loved an audience, singing songs on request for guests and doing hilarious imitations of family members. She was more confident; he was more easily hurt. Sometimes I didn't even realize I had slighted him until I glanced over and saw his blue eyes filling with tears. Meg might have asked me not to go, but such a request wouldn't have occurred to Tim. Putting off the kids' needs because of Don's was one thing, but was I justified in putting myself ahead of them too? By a fortunate coincidence, my in-laws were in town, staying at my sister-in-law's home, and I decided Tim would have plenty of people to care for him.

But I didn't feel good about leaving him. "What would a good mother do?" I asked myself. Would a good mother decide in favor of herself? My picture of a good mother didn't have a father with a wheelchair in it, though. When I came to a crossroads like this one, I had no role model. I never felt I had made the right choice, only the least hurtful to anyone, and sometimes not even that. I hated to think I might be neglecting my children.

Trying to fit everyone's needs into a twenty-four-hour day is, let's face it, impossible. Children's activities often occur at the end of an already exhausting day. Greta says that as Curt's ALS has worsened, she's become more involved in his care, and after an eight-hour workday of her own, she can hardly put one foot in front of the other. This is the first year she's had to miss some of the kids' activities, but she can't get off the treadmill. "I feel like we're really rigid in our schedule, there's just not a whole lot of flexibility. Anything extra, you pay the fiddler for. If I go to one of the kids' concerts, I'm up two hours later with Curt. I can never just go and do anything; there's always a price for it."

Yet paying that price may yield big dividends. "I sure tried to make things happen for them," says Diane Maxwell, speaking of outside activities for her sons. "That was a real sacrifice for me at times, because there were times when Jim had to be at the doctor, Tyler had to be on the football field, and Corey had to be at the bowling league." Diane accomplished this trick of being three places at once by calling on friends who had said, "Call me if I can do anything." "I called them and they were so thankful I asked for help." Encouraging and attending kids' activities is worth the effort, she believes, because "it says to the kids, you're important too, and your needs are important, and if this is important to you, we'll work on it." We, too, were blessed with neighbors and relatives who invited the kids on ski trips and other outings. Besides raising kids' self-esteem, sports and other activities build a sense of identity separate from having a sick parent. Just like us, kids need to feel effective in other areas of their lives, because we all feel helpless against the illness. The self-esteem that comes from activities can help considerably in keeping a parent's illness in perspective.

It's great if people offer to help, especially with kids, but most of the time, they aren't aware of our needs unless we make them known. We have no right to complain about the world's indifference if we haven't made the effort to ask. Did you know what it was like to be a well parent before you became one? Your neighbors still don't.

As the stress level in the household increases, emotions intensify. Adolescence is an angry time for kids anyway, but as Greta has found with Sandy, kids fight with the well parent because it's safe. They feel too guilty or afraid to take out their hostilities on a sick father or mother, so the well parent gets a double dose. "Emily, who was fourteen at the time, would vent her anger on me," says Kas Enger. "I remember one evening she was yelling and screaming at me about being too easy on her, and I needed to make her more responsible, and make her do things. I said, 'Wait a minute. Let me get this straight. I'm sitting in my own home being yelled at by my own daughter because I'm too easy on her. What's wrong with this picture?' We got her into counseling, and she seems to be past her horrible anger stage."

Helping children handle anger is one of the most important tools we give them. A child who is chronically angry may be overburdened by household and caregiving tasks, and may need the load lightened; this is where regular talks help. Tim inherited his dad's flashpoint temper, and I was frightened when, at age eight or nine, he shoved Don, who was standing precariously in his walker. Don tottered and almost fell. I took up the problem with my counselor, who was equally concerned. I had to take a firm stand on physical violence because, she said, "If he really hurt Don, think of the guilt he'd have to live with." She advised me to tell Tim that I understood he was angry, saying, "Everyone gets angry, and it's OK for you to be angry, but we don't hit other people." I came up with the idea of having the kids take a baseball bat to the wheelchair ramp in the garage when they got mad, and occasionally Don and I listened to the thumps and whacks of wood on wood. But they learned how to deal with anger, and now, at twenty and twenty-three, they are not angry adults.

Jake admits that his wife, in addition to being demanding, "had a reservoir of rage roiling just beneath the surface which would erupt without notice." He says, "I didn't know what the hell to do, so I escaped to my office and put in long hours." When Jake did come home in the evening he had a couple of drinks and tuned out. Eventually, the family was so out of control that all four went into family counseling. Jake's older son, Rick, "was old enough that he understood the value of it and cooperated with his therapist, eventually finding ways to resolve his fear, guilt, and anger." Rick joined the army after high school, and Jake believes it was to get away from the constant pain of seeing his mother suffer. His younger son, Doug, was another matter. "He fought counseling every step of the way, wouldn't cooperate, and lied to his therapist, and to me as well, about drinking, drugs, and sex." To Jake's despair, Doug was smart enough to con his therapist into thinking he was going along with the program, and then do exactly as he pleased. Things went from bad to worse when Doug ran away from home with his druggy friends. Jake was beside himself with fear and worry. One day, Jake happened to be at home when Doug came by to pick up some of his things, and he called the police. He had Doug arrested and committed to a psychiatric hospital for six weeks. After many bitter discussions, Jake agreed to let Doug get his own apartment while finishing high school. "He never came home," Jake concludes, "and didn't resolve his rage about his mom and me until after he got physical distance from us by leaving the state to go to college."

Yet today, as adults, Rick and Doug "are very caring people," Jake says. Rick takes care of his mom when he's home on leave from the army, and Doug—to Jake's surprise and gratification—is getting his master's degree in social work, and stays overnight with his mother so that Jake can take occasional trips. Despite his wife's continuing decline, Jake concludes, "At least one chapter in our family history has a happy ending."

It's easy to blame ourselves for not being super-parents in spite of the staggering challenges chronic illness brings. Sometimes we need to step back and remind ourselves that, life being what it is, our children might have had the same problems even with two healthy parents. I will always feel guilty about some things my children missed. Would my son's grades have been better if I'd spent more time with him? Would he have chosen to go to college right after high school, which I consider a necessity in our complex world, instead of getting a job? Now he owns a small restaurant, and my daughter is a nurse. They're law-abiding, responsible citizens, and I'm proud of them. If they're a bit hyper-mature, and take life a bit too seriously, I chalk it up to the cost of seeing their dad disintegrate before their eyes, and losing him so young—Tim was sixteen and Meg nineteen when he died. I won-der if I should have taken them on more vacations—just the three of us. I worry that they don't have enough fun in life, and then I realize that I'd much rather have them more responsible, than less. I know that even if Don hadn't been ill, I would have made mistakes in raising them. All living, but especially living the life of a well spouse, is a lesson in forgiving yourself. Well spouses do their best in crazy circumstances, and that's all that can be expected. I know that in some ways my children are better people because of Don, more compassionate, less self-centered. They have a more balanced picture of the world than kids who were raised to be the center of attention. Their knowledge of life's unfairness is, like so many things about this experience, both good and bad.

In trying to raise children with as few scars as possible, it's a good rule to save yourself first. Just as in an airplane parents are told to put on their own oxygen masks before tending to their children, so keeping ourselves mentally healthy is the best thing we can do for our children, because they will model their behav-ior on ours. Getting regular counseling helped me get timely intervention for my kids, as with Tim's anger. Because they saw Don and me getting help, they were willing to cooperate with family counselors during crises. Certainly, getting individual coun-seling for kids before small problems develop into big ones is essential. My children's junior high offered a support group for kids who had lost a parent or had one who was terminally ill, and my son attended that for a while. Interestingly, both children, on their own initiative, formed close friendships with other children who had lost a parent.

Sex educators talk about being an "askable" parent, and with a serious illness, we must model the same "askability" about the illness, because what kids imagine is a hundred times worse than the truth, no matter how grim. Children have fears surrounding an illness that would never occur to our adult minds. One day Don and I were discussing an article we had read about the mercury in silver fillings causing MS, a theory that was in vogue at the time. Tim, who had just gotten his first filling, overheard our conversation and was terrified he was about to get MS. After I reassured him, I thought how smart kids are, and how easily we forget that their minds, and their ears, are always working. I promised myself to be more sensitive in the future.

Cathy Rammelsberg says her daughters taught her the value of open communication. The oldest one began to confide in a friend's mother, and one day the woman called Cathy and said the girl had heard Cathy say David would have to go on dialysis, but the only part of "dialysis" she could make sense of was "die." Did dialysis mean her dad was going to die? Cathy called a huddle and explained that the procedure would save their dad, not kill him. Sometimes the three girls would overhear her explaining their father's condition to someone else, and complain that she "told people on the phone but not them." So Cathy began to keep them better informed.

Talking to our children isn't just a way to exchange information; it's a way to involve them in the ongoing problem-solving the illness requires. Whenever possible, tailoring the task to the child, so that he or she feels helpful but not oppressed, is a good idea. Josie Rammelsberg, Cathy's middle daughter, believes, "Each kid can do what he feels comfortable with." She had helped her dad butcher cows on their farm before he got kidney disease, so, she says, "I didn't mind doing dad's dressings. I always wanted to see his wounds, and know all about the procedures." When our children help, no matter how small the task, we must remember to praise and thank them. Knowing that they're contributing boosts their self-esteem and is a way of reminding them they're good, even if the situation is bad.

A parent learns to tread a delicate line between telling kids what's going on and giving them details that are too frightening or graphic. Let the children ask questions if they really want to know more. Cathy Rammelsberg says she drew the line at crying in front of her daughters. "One day I came in the back door and went to the basement," she says. "I was crying from exhaustion, but it scared them half to death. I don't know if they thought he had died, or what. I realized I couldn't do that again. I was the only one left standing, and I had to be strong."

"Being strong," however, may mislead children into thinking their own feelings of sadness and anger are bad or abnormal. While children who see their parents cry may temporarily feel a little less secure ("Mommy's crying, the world must be coming to an end"), hearing a parent express his or her own feelings reassures kids that their feelings are normal—and that it's safe to express them. The home is the place where children try out new behaviors and learn how to handle them. Maintaining that safe environment, especially when a sick parent lives there, is essential. Children growing up in this painfully uncertain situation need every reassurance, especially the security of knowing that they won't be loved any less, no matter what they do or say.

Another drawback to "being strong" is that kids take us at our word. For years, Barbara Beachman did all her husband's care without complaining, or asking any of their eight kids, Chuck's and hers, for help—emotional or practical. Barbara learned through a crisis to ask for help. Others may not learn this lesson until it's finally "safe" to fall apart, say, after the funeral, and then find themselves all alone, expected to be strong.

At the opposite and equally misguided extreme is turning a child into a confidant for a parent's worries. Kids deserve to be kids, and having to take on the added responsibility of consoling a well parent puts an unfair burden on slender shoulders. Well spouses need a strong support system—but of other adults, not their kids.

The truth is that children already worry about the healthy parent, more than we realize. I couldn't understand why Meg was so afraid to spend the night away from home, even as an adolescent, when most kids are delighted to escape their parents' clutches. I once had to order her onto a bus so that she and Tim could spend the weekend with my parents, to whom they were very close. I felt terribly guilty, even though I knew once she got there she would be fine. Only years later did it dawn on me—and her—that she was afraid something would happen to me while she was gone.

Always, children learn by example. A woman whose husband is seriously brain-injured has seen this principle in her own home. Two of her husband's daughter's sons, both three-year-olds, are afraid of him. But his son's two boys, ages three and four, "love their grandpa to pieces," she says. "I even have pictures of all three of my 'men' in their diapers!" she laughs. She sees her grandchildren mirroring their parents' attitudes. "If Howard's children are reluctant with their feelings, and have not faced their fears and losses, they can't expect any more from their own children," she concludes.

That so many of our children grow up to be well-adjusted adults is a tribute to their resilience, and is sometimes downright miraculous, considering what they've been through. John Hardin says, "I think my three children turned out very well. It's probably the thing I'm proudest of." Children who see us caring for sick partners learn a lesson stronger than words can teach. David Herndon says, "I feel like what I did in staying with Kay is a very significant model for my children. I cherish that today. . . . My kids have turned out well because I honored my commitment." Diane Maxwell reports, "I hear from teachers and church counselors and principals what great kids they are, over and over. It really validates that this whole illness is ugly, yet we can still be and still become good people in spite of it, or to spite it, maybe."

Looking back, Josie Rammelsberg reflects, "My dad's illness was pretty evenly divided between negative and positive stuff. It brought us closer, because my sisters and mom were the only people who understood what was going on. So if we ever needed to talk to somebody, we talked to each other." Happily, Josie's dad had a kidney transplant and has been able to resume his role of father.

Like Josie, my children are ambivalent when they look back on their father's illness. "Dad couldn't do all the father-son stuff, like playing catch and going to movies," said Tim, "so we didn't have the chance to bond together. I don't feel like I got to know him very well." As for good effects, "Dad's illness made me more mature than my friends. In high school, I wasn't into doing wild things. I guess I didn't really see the point of it." He smiles. "It kept me out of trouble."

Megan had some advice for other kids. "Understand that everything you feel is OK. I remember when one of our counselors said, 'Megan, do you want to tell your dad how you're feeling?' She had me tell Dad that I wished he would die, so he could be out of his pain. I loved him and loved who he was, and it was so hard. So, even wishing a parent would die, that's OK." She says, "It taught me to accept adversity in my life now, because dealing with Dad's illness was so hard. A parent's illness is bad and it's good, in that it teaches you to live each day, and not live with regrets."

# 8. Spirituality: "What Kind of God Could Do This?"

*Wearisome comforters are you all!*
*Is there no end to windy words?*
*Or what sickness have you that you speak on?*
*I also could talk as you do,*
*    were you in my place.*        —JOB 16:2–4

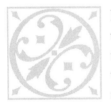 Every well spouse can identify with Job's frustration. The need to find causes and explanations where there are none makes fools of the wisest counselors, who are only too eager to rush in and advise us. However, as Job saw, finding meaning must be a personal journey.

A chronic illness forces us to ask the big questions. Finding meaning in suffering is one of the challenges, as well as one of the opportunities, of being a well spouse. Most of us discover that a belief system that served us well in the "before time" isn't enough when we try to make sense of what's happened, like a coat that fit in childhood but doesn't cover one's knees as an adult. Clergy who had a hot line to heaven before our spouses got sick find that the line is dead when we ask for help understanding the unexpected turn our lives have taken. Chronic illness, to quote poet Karl Shapiro, "cancels our metaphysics with a sneer."

Finding a mature spirituality was a task I wrestled with throughout Don's illness. When I was in the throes of some heartbreak in high school—an office I hadn't been elected to, a breakup with a boyfriend (how nostalgic those tragedies seem now)—my mother would tell me that "everything happens for the best." Usually time proved her right. But how could anything about Don's illness be "for the best," when everything about it was the worst? None of the bromides began to cover the enormity of this disaster. Even my mother couldn't find a silver lining for this one.

Not that friends stopped trying to find one. Roberta and I had become friends when I worked at the public library. I didn't know her well when Don was diagnosed, but I found her humorous, forthright way of looking at the world appealing, and we sometimes got together outside work. One day when I confessed how worried I was about the future, she told me she was a member of a fundamentalist group that believed God would heal people whose faith was sufficient. If Don believed strongly enough in his own healing, he would be cured. "I hate to see people settling for bad health," she said. "He doesn't have to have MS." She admonished me not to give in to the disease. "Believe for a miracle, and it will happen."

I left her apartment with my head spinning. How could she call herself my friend? I had no idea what she was talking about, for one thing. My husband had a strong belief in God. And he was so moral that, long before he got a crippling illness, he had written off one of our favorite restaurants because they refused to admit handicapped people. The idea that he was choosing to stay sick with MS made me furious. No one wanted to be healed more than he did. On the other hand, I had to wonder if there was any merit to her thinking. Could Don pray himself back to health? I had heard of miraculous healings, but had read that they were the result of hysteria, not faith. Was Roberta's faith really faith, or naivete? If wishing one's way out of disease was so easy, no one would be sick. Roberta was my first contact with religion as bludgeon.

If only the universe were as just as she made it sound, you could trade in your sickness as easily as you'd return a pair of shoes. "Excuse me, I didn't order this. I'd like a refund." I had taken only the required biology and physical science classes in college, but even that little bit of science had taught me that life-forms obeyed certain laws as they competed for space and food. Viruses and bacteria, though lowly, had equal entitlement with the higher forms. Sometimes they beat us to the trough. That we had consciousness and imagination and emotions and souls didn't signify in this war. And our gifts didn't necessarily help us overcome our microscopic brethren. Furthermore, the God I was familiar with didn't jump at anyone's beck and call. Even when he at last spoke to Job, he didn't explain himself. As the creator of the universe, he allowed physics and biology to work; that's why they were called laws.

I understood why illnesses like Don's begged for explanations. What could bring more primal terror than the thought that a young healthy person could go to bed one night and the next morning be unable to move? You're going along thinking life can only get better, and suddenly you're paralyzed. To admit that such catastrophes can happen without warning to any of us makes our orderly little worlds feel definitely disordered. We feel panicky, out of control, at the realization that we are minuscule beings in a huge, chaotic universe. We strive to regain the sense of a plan, that things happen for a reason. When nothing else presents itself, we figure the person himself must have provoked the illness. In this way, we're still cave dwellers in our search for answers. Just as primitive people explained catastrophes by saying that the gods must be angry, modern people, in spite of the sophistries of medicine, look for similar explanations. Don and I were no exception. What had we done to anger the gods? What misstep, what sin of omission or commission, what mortal or venial sin or combination thereof was Don guilty of? For my part, I couldn't help wondering what sinister transaction had occurred between my husband and his God and the devil before I arrived on the scene.

As Susan Sontag has noted, illness in America has moral implications. Our sophistication about the cause of certain diseases has led to a kind of hubris. A victim of lung cancer is assumed to have been a smoker; of liver disease, a drinker; of AIDS, an indiscriminate sex partner. When none of these applies, we resort to more esoteric reasons. "Dis-ease," in new-age healthspeak, is a malady we bring on ourselves because of some conflict we didn't deal with efficiently in the past. Blaming the victim has the advantage of a flesh-and-blood target. Admitting that we don't know makes us feel helpless and dumb. Acquaintances tried these theories out on me sometimes. "Mary thinks she got MS because she (couldn't forgive her sister; was in a bad marriage; was under stress at work)." I tried to keep the heat out of my voice when I replied, "No one knows what causes MS." I was comforted to find this statement in Sontag's *Illness as Metaphor:* "Theories that diseases are caused by mental states and can be cured by will power are always an index of how much is not understood about the physical terrain of a disease." And what disease was more terra incognita than multiple sclerosis?

Then, in spite of myself, I went home and thought about why Don had gotten MS. Try as I might, I could think of nothing of sufficient gravity. The oldest of four, Don had a happy childhood, with adoring parents and a sizable extended family. As for holding grudges or nursing hostilities, my husband was someone who flared up quickly but forgave just as fast. He had a confidence about his place in the world, in the gentle way of big men, who know they don't have to raise their voices to be heard. He was one of the most balanced people I'd ever known. Only someone who didn't know him would believe he had attracted his MS.

Of greater seriousness was his mother's mental illness. When Don was in high school, Margaret had a serious mental break-down, and spent months in a psychiatric hospital. Her depression was so bad she was given electroshock treatments, and in those days, they deserved their horror-movie reputation. "She was never the same after that," Don once wept. Her memory problems, a result of the shock treatments, blighted the rest of her life.

So his life had been touched by real trauma, but the family had come through intact. His grandmother, Josie, a tiny Irish-woman who favored wearing black, came to live with them during that time, and while she was peppery and uncompromising in her rules, she kept the family together. And Don genuinely loved her.

I scanned the recent past. We had bought our first house less than a year before his symptoms appeared. But he was proud as a lord of our modest, newly constructed three-bedroom ranch house. Maybe his new job? But he loved his work, and was good at it. Our marriage was happy, and our two little blond chil-dren were glowingly healthy. In some ways, we were the picture-perfect American family.

The corollary to the he-must-have-brought-it-on-himself the-ory is this: We'll forgive you for being sick as long as you're getting better. The media loves stories of people overcoming handicaps and illnesses, implying that if you're not getting better, you're not trying hard enough. Americans are goal-oriented, with illness as with everything else. Attitude is everything. If it doesn't keep us from getting sick in the first place, it can certainly cure us. People didn't know what to say to someone with a chronic illness that only worsened. Like Job's friends, they were exasperated by a disease that wouldn't yield to the usual remedies. While I shifted from foot to foot, acquaintances—and sometimes total strangers, stopped in their tracks by the sight of a young man in a wheelchair—brought out stories of relatives or friends cured by bee venom, macrobiotic diets, electric shock devices. Anyone with chronic illness gets used to these recitations, with their implied message. For the religiously inclined, if not even God, the court of last resort, was helping here, then the fault must be the victim's own recalcitrance. His faith must not be strong enough. I loved the story I heard about a recent widow who encountered a friend in the grocery store. Her husband was ill, the friend said, but "he's going to recover—we're Christian, you know."

Spouses, on the other hand, get different reactions. Mostly we're invisible. We get used to members of the medical profession looking past us in order to check the condition of the patient. We learn quickly that it's the sick person who counts, not the person behind the wheelchair. In public, people ask, "How's Don doing?" or "How's Betty?" rather than "How are you?" One woman said she was going to have a T-shirt printed that said, "He's fine! Don't ask!"

But sometimes being noticed feels worse, because the attention takes another, equally discomfiting form—hero worship. I've referred to this phenomenon earlier as the "plaster saint syndrome" the world wants to immobilize us with. "You're so brave! I could never do what you do!" we're told in the grocery store, in church, in the doctor's office. We can be excused for feeling schizoid in these situations. We know only too well the unsaintly thoughts that sometimes cross our minds. As one wife said, "I'd be holding on to his wheelchair at the top of the stairs and find myself thinking, 'just one little push.'" Far from feeling angelic, most of us doubt that we still inhabit the same benevolent universe as the rest of the world. Maggie Strong, founder of the Well Spouse Foundation, writes that sometimes when she is speaking before groups she is asked whether she doesn't find it spiritually uplifting to care for another human being. She hesitates before answering, uncomfortably aware of the expectations of the audience before replying, "No, I don't." We'd settle for feeling human most days.

The question of faith kept intruding. At Don's parents' urging, we visited a young couple they knew from church. The wife had had MS for two years. Leaning on her husband and her cane, she wobbled over to the sofa, but we were about to find out that there was nothing tentative about her beliefs. She began to talk about her illness, how it had started, how her family, a husband and teenage daughter and son, rearranged their routines to help her. Reaching for the Bible on the coffee table, she opened it to a purple bookmark. Her quavering voice grew stronger as she got to the last line: "By his stripes I am healed." She stared at us, jabbing her finger at the book. "It's right here in Isaiah. By his stripes I am healed." She continued more emphatically. "I know I'm going to get well, because Jesus Christ died for me. I will be healed of my MS because of him."

"Are you sure that means physical healing?" I ventured hesitantly. "Yes," she insisted. "He told us to ask and we shall receive. If we ask anything in His name, He will give it to us. I will be healed."

If faith is a requisite for healing, I thought, this woman is due for a miracle. I wondered if God would rise to the occasion.

Don's parents seemed to think these encounters with fellow sufferers would help us soldier on, comforted that we were not alone. But when I left the Bible-believer, I was depressed and full of questions. She was like Roberta in her stridency, but was she professing faith or superstition? She had backed herself into a cor-

*[handwritten in margin: Faith, God, man & miracles?]*

ner, made herself another prison in addition to her illness. It seemed a risky proposition to me, daring God to heal you. I understood how MS could drive someone to that extreme, but I was afraid for her. I wished I had had the eloquence to explain that faith means believing in God, not necessarily miracles. I also knew that she wouldn't have listened. A few years later, we heard that her MS was much worse, and she no longer went to church.

Don and I were not above desperate measures ourselves. At our last visit to the neurologist, he had parting words for us: He seldom saw a case as relentless as Don's. When Dr. Shepard told us that chemotherapy was being tried on MS patients as a way to kill off some of the white cells destroying the myelin sheath that insulated the nerves, we decided to try it. With high hopes, Don checked himself into the hospital on our daughter's ninth birthday. He believed in these little signs. But after five days of unremitting vomiting, he gave up the therapy. I had never seen him so depressed. His stay in the hospital seemed to have burned away his hope as well as his blood cells. A few months later, when my mother mentioned that Father Ralph Diorio was coming to Great Falls, we were willing to consider it.

Stories of miraculous healings followed the Catholic priest like a vapor trail. Some had people throwing away their crutches or abandoning their wheelchairs after he had laid hands on them. I mentioned the event to Don, and like me, he felt he had nothing to lose. On a clear October evening I pushed his wheelchair after the ushers to the front row of an enormous arena, next to the stage. The bleachers were full to the top. I looked out at the sea of wheelchairs, awed at the suffering that had brought each of them here. I felt strangely at home, but as we waited for the priest to appear, Don leaned toward me. "I always scorned those Oral Roberts programs. Now I'm at one. Complete with its own freak show." His eyes filled.

*165*

During the program, the priest left the stage and prayed over those who were coming forward in long lines. As the numbers dwindled, he turned to those nearest the stage. He spotted Don and began to walk toward him. Laying his hands on Don's head he prayed inaudibly, only his lips moving. I scarcely dared to breathe. Was this our miracle at last? We had been looking for it in the bottom of an IV bag, but maybe it was in the hands of this kind-faced, rotund cleric.

The priest finished and turned away. I was afraid to look at Don. But nothing happened. He didn't stand up and walk.

In the car he said wonderingly, "It happened exactly the way I pictured it, that he would see me in the crowd, and walk over to me." Except, I couldn't bring myself to say, you aren't healed. It didn't happen. Instead I said, "There are lots of different kinds of healing. Maybe you got a kind we can't see." I was relieved that he seemed to agree with this. Then, I wouldn't have been able to explain what I meant.

Some spouses find that, like certain friends, their churches are supportive only when the sun is shining. Barbara Beachman had to get rid of her church in order to find God. She and her husband Chuck's lives had centered around their fundamentalist, evangelical church, which believed in faith healing. Initially, they tried that method, but when it didn't work, Chuck became embittered. She was disappointed too, but not enough to lose her faith. "You think, 'OK, Lord, I've lived this good life. Why is this happening?' And you've got to go on from that." Church members criticized her for caving in. "They told me, 'You shouldn't admit that he has MS.' And I'd say, 'But this is what he has.' And they'd say, 'But you've got to speak out in faith that he's been healed.' Well, forget that." Their idea of faith was her idea of denial. She decided she could deal with God, but not with the censure of those who were supposed to reflect God's love for her and Chuck.

She claims she feels closer to God now, but doesn't go to any particular church.

Pat Oswald had a similar experience. She describes their former church, a Church of Religious Science, as "new age." She remembers, "Here Fran was, on a respirator, and they would say things like, 'You brought this on yourself' and 'When you make up your mind to get well, you will.' This went on for two or three months, and finally I asked them not to come back." Pat complained that such visits weren't helpful, but the minister seemed unconcerned. About three years into Fran's illness, a neighbor invited Pat to attend her church. "This was the most wonderful church," Pat says. "Fran and I didn't even belong, but the minister came so many times to see Fran. There were three assistant ministers, and they all came to see him. Every Sunday they brought him communion. They were even at his memorial service. The support from that church was phenomenal."

For Bob Keller, the lack of caring from clergy has left him permanently soured on Catholicism. "Spiritual counseling would have been a big help five or six years ago," he says. "I don't know that it would help now. I've gotten through the worst part." He is particularly angry at the pastor of his and Ellen's parish. "He knew what kind of condition she was in," he complains. "I don't think he ever went up to the nursing home. Why can't he do that? He's a priest." He shakes his head angrily. Bob still attends church, though not the one he attended with Ellen. "I wouldn't go out and recruit anyone to join the Catholic Church," he says. "Call me a disillusioned Catholic."

As these people found out, churches are run by human beings with varying degrees of compassion. Watching someone die slowly shakes the foundations of our faith, and when our churches desert us, too, we may be hard-pressed to find our way back to God.

If that's where we want to go. We may feel like Barbara

Beachman: "OK, Lord, I've lived this good life. Why is this happening?" Or as Margy Kleinerman wrote despairingly to her rabbi: "My husband has Alzheimer's and has been in a nursing home for the last year. He has other physical problems in addition to this devastating disease. He was a former college professor, fluent in six languages. He is only seventy-two years old. Although we belong to a Reform temple, he would lay Tefillin every morning, would not eat seafood or pork. He was certainly prayerful, repentant, and charitable, giving generously to both Jewish and non-Jewish charities. He was a very devoted family man. Now I watch him deteriorate, and I wonder what kind of God can do this to such a good person."

*What kind of God can do this to such a good person?* The question echoes, as unanswerable now as it was in Job's time.

Some have an easier time with acceptance than others. When I commented to Bill Hill, who cares for his wife at home, that he seemed so serene, whereas I had so much anger when Don was sick, he smiled and shrugged. "I don't have it because I've had more life than you have. I'm older than you are." And Paul Kleffner says, "I'm not angry. All I have to do is look a little further, and I see someone with a bigger problem than mine. I feel really blessed in spite of this little cross to bear."

David Herndon's wife, Kay, was forty-three when she got Parkinson's. "What happened to Kay is not so bad when you view what happens daily in our society as far as people are concerned," he says. "There's a lot of cruel reality in human experience, like child abuse and crime. There are worse evils than illnesses like Kay's. I really don't have a quarrel with God about what happened."

Others are not so philosophical. Roy Layton's frustration that his prayers were not answered made him abandon his faith—in his own ability to keep a commitment that meant so much to him, and in his God. He and Donna were devout Mormons, and as the demands of her illness increased, Roy turned to church elders for guidance. "They profess that God is interested in people's welfare. If people express their needs through prayer, they will get some kind of resolution, some kind of answer, some kind of understanding of their situation," he says. He continues, "Our prayers were not being answered. Instead I saw Donna get worse, my work get harder, and my understanding of it get less and less. Finally I threw it all out in disgust." Of his spirituality now, he says, "I don't think I'm an atheist, because an atheist believes there is no God. And I don't think I'm agnostic, because an agnostic is somebody that says wait and see. I would say I'm a cynic. If there is a God, he's a mean one."

Even if asking why is not particularly profitable, it's hard not to if we believed, in our previous lives, that God would deal with us fairly. We thought if we lived good lives, went to church, didn't hurt people, and paid our taxes, nothing bad would happen to us. Evil was theoretical, and mostly something that happened to other people. Personal tragedy destroys these cozy illusions. We see that our beliefs were superstition, not faith. We know ourselves to be innocent of any offense that would have brought this kind of wrath. Or do we?

Hilde struggled with this idea after Hank's accident. "I thought maybe there was something I needed to atone for. I thought God was doing this to me for a reason. I thought it might be because I wasn't a good enough person, and now I have to pay for this. I truly believed that." Her parish priest helped her to remember all the compassionate things she had done in her life and to accept that she was not being punished. She arrived at what was for her a better dynamic. "There aren't too many people who go straight to heaven," she says. "I believe you somehow have to cleanse yourself. You have to go to purgatory before you can see the face of God in heaven. I yak a lot to God." She laughs. "I say, 'You take that off,' if I have a bad day or something. I say, 'This ought to count for something, a couple of days or something.' My priest says, 'Hilde, you'll go straight to heaven!'" Another woman, whose husband is in a nursing home with Parkinson's, says, "I think God is doing all of this to make me stronger." She pauses. "I think I do. I don't know."

In facing a partner's mortality we face our own. Maintaining faith in some kind of benevolent power in the teeth of this daily slide toward entropy is a huge challenge; still, we can't bring ourselves not to. Therese Rando, a thanatologist, has said that "pain is suffering without meaning." Well spouses need to believe that suffering, ours and our partners', has meaning beyond the day-to-day; otherwise, the pointlessness adds another layer of pain. One woman who cares for her husband with MS at home says: "If it wasn't for my spiritual life, I wouldn't make it. I know that God is in control. I don't know why, but I have to believe he's in charge." She starts to cry. "God wouldn't do this if there weren't some good in it someplace. For the most part, I can't see it. But it hasn't shaken my faith." Knowing we've made the right choice would be reassuring, but those who search for a sign are doomed to disappointment, as Linda Anderson discovered. "I wanted to know why Steve was getting worse. I wasn't getting any answers, and I was really ticked about that. Finally, after weeks of feeling angry and guilty and wondering why this was continuing in my life, I realized it's a matter of trust. It's called faith for a reason, because there are rarely physical signs."

Deanne Foley, whose husband, Carl, has ALS, says, "I don't know how people deal with this without faith. Where do they get any peace?" She says that it took her a "long, long time" to come to grips with why God allowed Carl's illness. She says, "This is not God's desire for Carl and our family. His desire is the Garden of Eden. The reason that there is suffering is that we live in a world that has free choice, and because of that there is evil and there is illness. And somehow he must just step back and give us that free choice. For him to intervene, that would take free choice from us. Those are the things that have given me peace." She adds, "I guess I'm learning a lot about trust, and learning to lay all these things at the foot of the Cross, and just saying, 'You are in control. . . . I don't get the big picture, but I trust you to do with this what you will.' "

Sometimes, that degree of trust only comes after a dark night of the soul. Kas Enger's husband, Ken, had had MS for seven years when her oldest daughter, Michael Ann, was diagnosed with it at age fifteen. "Somehow," Kas says, "I had it in my mind that God only allows one bad thing per person. Or per couple. I don't know where I got that, but sort of subconsciously, that's what I thought. So when my daughter was diagnosed, that blew my belief out of the water. I was very, very angry with God." Slowly, she says, she realized that God already knew she had the anger in her heart, so why not yell at him and tell him so? "So I did a lot of yelling at him." Gradually the yelling turned to praying, and like Deanne Foley, Kas began to trust again. "I have just had to rely on prayer and on my faith that God is going to bring good out of this somehow."

Donna Keefe's husband, Pat, told her that he could feel her praying for him while he was on a respirator and unconscious after extensive, and very dangerous, surgery. Even though Donna was more than six hundred miles away at the time, she says that "he knew there was a force of some kind." And Mark and Bonnie Johannes's shared faith has helped keep them together. "We pray together, every night, out loud. It helps our marriage," says Mark.

There are spiritual rewards to being a well spouse, but the full bedpans and empty checkbook can obscure them. The day-to-day detritus of chronic illness prevents us from seeing the big picture, that of helping another person live. Buddhists believe no one gets into heaven who hasn't brought someone else along; we know we're doing just that, even if we may not articulate it in that way, or articulate it at all. Christians have the model of the god/man who redeemed the world with his suffering: "There is no greater love than this: to lay down one's life for one's friends" (John 15:13). All Christians are called by his example, but well spouses have the opportunity to be visible examples of the lesson of the Cross. Jesus himself exhibited the confusion and doubt and despair and anger that are part of following God's will. Even he, on the eve of the Crucifixion, prayed, "If it be thy will, let this cup pass away. But not my will, but thine, be done." Nowhere in the Bible does God promise us an easy life. What he did promise was that he would always be with us, "even to the end of the world."

The suffering on the Cross led to the world's redemption, but do our crosses lead to some kind of redemption? This question is at the center of the mystery, and Americans are impatient with mystery. "What does it mean?" I kept asking myself. "What does my sacrifice mean?" I wanted immediate, quantifiable results, beyond my husband's gratitude, beyond providing a good example for my children. After Don went to the nursing home in 1988 I felt especially lost. I felt guilty that I couldn't care for Don at home anymore, confused about my status (was I wife or widow?), and constantly worried about the future. Then I read a newspaper article about Marietta Jaeger. Marietta was vacationing in Montana in the summer of 1973 with her husband and five children. One night while the family slept in two adjacent tents, her seven-year-old daughter, Susie, was taken by a man who cut a neat square in the side of one of the tents and lifted her through it.

Against all expectations, the crime became a spiritual turning point for her. I called her and asked if I could interview her for an article.

Through a supreme act of will, she told me, she decided after Susie's disappearance to begin praying for her abductor. On the anniversary of the crime, to the exact minute, he called to taunt her—and to admit that he had murdered her daughter. During their hour-long conversation, he gave away enough information that the FBI was able to trace and arrest him. He eventually confessed to raping and strangling Susie, then incinerating her body. Marietta, though grief stricken, continued to pray for David Meirhofer. In one phone conversation, she told him she forgave him. Over time, she found, to her surprise, that she truly did feel forgiveness for him, and prayed that he would find peace. She was stunned when word came that he had hanged himself in jail before he could be tried. Searching for closure, she traveled from Detroit to Montana to pray in his empty cell. As she knelt there that afternoon, the dingy jail came to symbolize the prison she and David and Susie found themselves in. David had been a prisoner of his own evil compulsions, and she and Susie had been caught in that evil web by time and circumstance. Kneeling on the dirty floor, crushed by the sadness and horror of the past year, she saw the cell walls suddenly light up, their ugliness transformed into something otherworldly. Blinking in surprise, she believed it was God's message that her and David's odyssey, filled with violence and despair, was touched with grace. In the following months, she began speaking to groups on the power of forgiveness, and became an eloquent opponent of the death penalty.

I realized why Marietta had come into my life then. Our circumstances were quite different, yet one of her statements came to me again and again. "God can redeem even the most horrible situation." Surely if she could keep believing in God's goodness through the murder of her child, I could find some good in my young husband's slow dying. I didn't realize until much later that Marietta's message of forgiveness spoke to me because I, too, and all well spouses, had something to forgive: the theft of my husband's life. Marietta taught me that seeing the good in tragedy requires a kind of vision that has nothing to do with eyes.

The need to find meaning from the well spouse experience can lead to deeper spirituality. A path that leads down and down to a partner's humiliating death, and the waste of our own time and talents, doesn't offer any peace. Much as we don't want to be seen as examples, we are. Much as we wish we could read a book and learn these lessons, we can't. The Native Americans have a saying: "The hard road and the easy road sometimes cross. And where they do, the ground is holy." Finding the holiness on this hard road is a necessity if we are not to suffer needlessly. I suspect this search is why well spouses stay. Somehow we realize that this experience has something to teach us that we will not learn any other way. Finding meaning in it feels all the more pressing because it relentlessly defies us to find good in it anywhere.

Recognizing that every life is a precious gift from the Creator makes us ask ourselves what God expects of us. We look at the array of gifts and talents that make us uniquely who we are, and ask: Is being a caregiver, and only a caregiver, my highest purpose in life? Is this all God wants from me? I couldn't believe that. I came to believe that I had a duty to God to develop other aspects of myself, which would be possible only if I had a life apart from caregiving, one that allowed me to become the person he had made me to be. I could not believe that a good and loving God expected me, or any of his creatures, to be miserable.

Occasionally our spouses inspire us. Fran Oswald's helplessness, says Pat, "made him trust God more. He told me it made him closer to God." She saw the results of that closeness in his acceptance of some painful realities. "He resolved things with his children, in the sense that he resolved that it was unresolvable. Any old business he and I had, that was totally resolved." For Pat and Fran, and for many believers, death was the healing they had prayed for.

Many well spouses speak of discovering the strength that lies within. "I've gotten a lot of good out of this," says Debbie Lang. "I've learned how to research the illness and find help where I can. And I'm learning what I can and can't handle." Natalie says, "I've been able through therapy to become a different person than I was, and to learn what's acceptable to me and what's not. If I'm going to be in this relationship, I'm going to make it the best it can possibly be. I'm not happy about how I got here, but I like the person I've become."

A man whose wife has had MS for twenty years says, "Through a seven-year process of individual and group therapy, I eventually met this new person whom I liked—myself. A brick had been transformed magically into a flowering tree who could be strong and yet also feel and express his soft side."

Pam Cook, whose husband is brain-damaged from a workplace accident, says, "I've learned patience where it's needed, assertiveness when it's necessary, and the ability to love and find good, even in bad situations. You don't have to be miserable."

Whether we like it or not, we provide the rest of the world with a living example that love is sacrifice. It's hard to imagine that emptying a catheter bag is mirroring God's love. But it is.

Our children are the primary beneficiaries of our example, and many well spouses find that their children turn into unusually empathic adults as a result of the caring they saw demonstrated daily at home. We would never have wished it on them, but who can deny the profound lessons in love they learned growing up in our homes?

Our own suffering makes us aware, as never before, of the suffering of others. The idea that our influence on others' lives doesn't end with our lives, or even with theirs, but stretches outward in widening circles, in ways we cannot imagine, is a hopeful one. Linda Anderson has seen good come from her suffering. "I firmly believe that no experience is ever wasted. Everything can be used. If I thought that what I went through the last fifteen to sixteen years meant nothing, I would be in despair, but I do not believe that. It can have meaning. It has to do with being open to letting God use us as a tool in our lives. As a church secretary, I'm the first one people see. I can't tell you how many people ask me, can I run something past you? And I can't tell you how many phone calls I've gotten."

"Wounded healers," Henri Nouwen calls those whose suffering makes them uniquely equipped to minister to others. I was furious once when someone suggested that Don got MS so that I could grow spiritually. Nothing in this life, certainly not my spiritual growth, I assured this man, could ever justify my husband's suffering. But like other spouses here, I believe all human experience can be mined. In Therese Rando's framework, life may be painful, but it doesn't have to be meaningless pain.

"One of my students wrote a poem," says Eugenia Staerker. "It was 'God sends us Angels.' God can't come here in person, but he sends us other people. If well spouses reach out, they find people." Reaching out, admitting we don't know, admitting we can't do this alone, is a difficult first step, but it's one that must be taken if we are to survive and grow. Admitting that we're human like everyone else doesn't have to depress us; it can be a reminder that our humanity unites us in life-giving ways with everyone else on earth.

In our communities are other wounded healers, whose gifts may fit our needs now, just as our gifts someday may fit their needs. We never know, when we reach out, who will respond. Well spouses have been shocked to find others in their community who consider taking care of the sick a ministry that enriches their lives. Their need becomes another's gift. Many well spouses volunteer in their communities and churches. They participate in—and run—support groups not just for the help they get, but for the help they can give—even though they are heavily burdened themselves. Feeling connected reminds us that we're part of the circle of life, and this awareness can help us see beyond our own troubles.

# 9. Why Stay?: "Just Something That's in Me"

The vows we said as two healthy people, so romantic and ephemeral that bright summer day in a flower-bedecked church, sound like a prison sentence when one of us develops an intractable disease. "The problem with the words 'in sickness and in health,'" said one husband plaintively, "is that, when you say them, you think of the flu or something you recover from." The Catholic ceremony, as I recall, said something about the future being hidden from our eyes. Which was a good thing, I thought later, or I would have run screaming from the church.

Do people divorce because of illness? "There's not much good data, and there should be," says John Rolland, M.D., author of *Families, Illness, and Disability*, who explains that collecting information is complicated because other things besides illness figure into whether marriages break up. Tom Campbell, M.D., associate professor of family medicine and psychiatry at the University of Rochester, says, "We do know that people with chronic illness have much higher divorce rates. But the question is, what's the relationship? Does divorce cause chronic illness, or do health problems cause divorce? Or is some other factor causing both?"

Pam Cavallo, director of clinical programs at the National MS Society, says that a national study commissioned by the society in 1990 came up with the surprising finding that MS couples divorce less often than the general population. Eighty-five percent of the MS population was married, while only 62 percent of the general population was. For years, Don and I heard that 90 percent of marriages with MS fail. The 1990 study doesn't bear this out, and Cavallo denies that the 90 percent figure came from the MS Society.

Spouses may have an easier time leaving a troubled marriage if the partner is physically healthy and can care for himself. It's possible that, after illness hits, people who would have divorced feel too guilty to leave a sick husband or wife. So maybe in some cases, illness keeps couples together. Abandoning a sick person is a powerful social taboo, even for those who don't put much stock in traditional religion. One wife referred to this pressure as "fear of abandoning, rather than fear of abandonment."

Nevertheless, I have been surprised, in talking to spouses, at the commitment many expressed. A psychologist who counsels patients with chronic illness and their families, Susan Brace, R.N., Ph.D., says that in her experience, rarely do couples with chronic illness break up. She theorizes that they stay together partly because, right from the start, the illness is something they share, unlike a diving accident or car crash that happens suddenly. In her practice, accidents cause more marital breakups than illness. She explains, "Both of you realize something isn't right. You might not know what it is, you may actually nurse it along for a while, thinking you're making little changes and it's responding positively until you finally realize, we need to go see somebody." Often the spouses are together when they get the bad news. Bette Allbright, whose husband, Jim, is now in a nursing home, says, "I loved my husband and knew it would be for life, and with the disease, I knew it would be for life too."

What keeps us in marriages that no longer bear any resemblance to the ones we once had? Don once told me that "this is harder for you because you have a choice." The concept that caregiving is a choice should be good news, but it only adds a psychological twist of the knife. Every day we face a situation that drives us to the wall. One husband spoke of his wife's supra-pubic catheter, a tube connecting her bladder to a catheter bag, as an improvement over an intermittent catheter bag because he doesn't have to change it as often. The disadvantage of the new method, however, is that it leads to more bladder infections. He says ruefully, "I have become satisfied with relative benefits because total resolution of problems is impossible. There are no victories in the war against chronic progressive MS—only an occasional and temporary retreat to a slightly better place with the understanding that your position will soon be overrun again by the enemy." This enemy is crueler than most, because it allows the victim to suffer for endless years without killing. I pictured Don's MS as a huge, malevolent beast that toyed with him till he was near death, then walked away until he recovered sufficiently for the next round. One wife said of her quadriplegic husband, "I'd get my hopes up when he had trouble breathing."

Why would any sane person stay in such a hell? It was a question I asked myself every day, and on an especially bad day, more than once. As Don said, I had a choice. And recognizing that I stayed voluntarily, that no thug was holding a gun to my head, made the question even harder to answer.

In spite of his remark, I didn't fully recognize that I had chosen to stay until a counselor pointed it out. I had been looking for part-time work, and my counselor asked me what I would say to a prospective employer about why my career as a college English teacher had languished. I replied, "I had to take care of my husband." She challenged me. "That's a powerless statement. Rephrase it so it reflects the choice you made to make a home for your husband and children, that that was an important value for you." I did, and a little light dawned that day. I understood for the first time that, as much as I felt I was being swept along by a raging current of love, guilt, obligation, and fear, at some point I had made a decision to stay, even if I had never thought of it as one.

Because we get sucked into caregiving so gradually, we don't realize we've made a decision. In a crisis, we have to act, and there's no one else to do it for us. You can't let your husband or wife lie there in the ruins of a potted plant, soiled with his or her own feces and urine. You can't refuse a shoulder to lean on or a ride to work. You can't refuse a cup of water to someone who's thirsty, or a plate of food to someone who's hungry. In addition to all the caregiving duties, you assume all the chores your partner can't do anymore. The needs escalate, and one day you realize you've become a full-time caregiver—and the sole caregiver at that. Kas Enger says, "Just because you're the marriage partner, you end up being the caregiver by default. Nobody asks, but everybody expects it." The notion that caregiving was a choice didn't dawn on her until Ken began to need home health aides. For Kas, the fact that "some people have chosen to do this for a living" was a revelation. Recognizing that she was choosing to do what some people consider a full-time job gave her a new sense of autonomy.

That insight hasn't compensated for the fact that she often feels like a slave. "He has this doorbell-type thing that you plug into an electric outlet, and there's a button on his motorized cart, and he has another button in the bathroom. So if he needs help, he rings," she says. "He never abuses it," she stresses. Neverthe-less, "I hate that button with a passion. When he rings that bell I just see visions of this little slave person being summoned." She dreads the bell because often when it rings it's because he's fallen, and although Ken weighs 160 pounds, "it feels like three hundred pounds of dead weight." Barbara Drucker says, "Sometimes I'd like to change my name. I mean, it's always Barbara, BARBARA! Sometimes I'll say, you're not going to die of natural causes because I'm going to kill you first."

"I envy the widows," one woman said, speaking the unspeak-able. We long for a blessed end to pain—theirs and ours—a peaceful death, a funeral, a time at last to mourn a life that never was. Instead, when we look ahead, we see only a cycle of draining days followed by sleepless nights that stretches into the horizon. One woman with health problems of her own confessed that she was "mad as hell" that her husband might outlive her.

The notion that caregiving is a choice takes us only so far. After all, as the burden gets heavier and heavier, why would any normal person keep choosing to stay? As one woman complained, "Choosing to be a full-time volunteer in your own life is an odd idea." My subconscious drew terrifying pictures at night. I'd wake up gasping because I dreamed that while I was sleeping, the bed-room ceiling had steadily descended until it was a few inches from my face. I was being buried alive! As year after year passed, with Don's condition steadily worsening, the idea that I had chosen this life, and continued to choose it, became a torment. Was I crazy for staying? What good was it doing? Had I become a pain junkie, or hopelessly "codependent," the buzzword of the eighties?

When Socrates said the unexamined life was not worth liv-ing, he must have had well spouses in mind, because I constantly found myself holding my tattered life up to the light, wondering why I was here. Illness made me ask the big questions. What does life mean? What does love mean? And the nagging, perpetually unanswerable one: What do I owe this person I've joined fates with?

Love, as well spouses discover, is a tender trap. For me, it was both the reason I stayed and the reason I could hardly bear to. I knew to an absolute certainty that I loved my husband; I knew it the way I knew my eyes were brown. That fact was hard to keep uppermost, but underneath it all, I knew that was why I stayed. Remarkably, Don kept his sense of humor, and kept loving us, too, and those things helped a lot. He could be demanding, but he was never emotionally or physically abusive. He thanked me for my efforts, and sometimes he apologized, saying, "I'm sorry I dragged you into this." The chief effect on his brain from the MS was emotional lability, which increased over time. Mostly, that meant he cried more easily. He never suffered the personality and cognitive changes some with MS do. That he remained, psychologically anyway, the man I married was a singular blessing, because unlike other well spouses whose partners are hostile and emotionally abusive, I don't know that I could have stayed otherwise.

Or was it a curse? Maybe, if he had become someone else, I could have stayed more comfortably. The fact that he remained my Don made watching him die slowly of MS a protracted agony.

I understood that the reason I hurt so much was because I loved so much. I wanted to hang on to spite the MS, to show it that it couldn't take everything. Even if it succeeded in killing my husband, it wouldn't have the last word. This conviction helped me maintain some sense of power in the face of constant, degrading losses.

In a similar way, when I thought about leaving, his courage gave me pause. Every day he hauled himself out of bed and, with the help of an aide, spent two hours getting toileted and dressed and shaved. He worked until he physically couldn't work anymore, and had to be asked to leave. How could I quit on someone who wouldn't quit on himself?

The literature I had studied in college and graduate school kept some important truths in front of me. The great writers often devoted their best work to the theme of human suffering, and one poem I studied as an undergraduate came to be especially meaningful. In "On Wenlock Edge," English poet A. E. Housman says that life is intense because it's so short. The poet, observing a thunderstorm raking the English countryside, reflects that this spot was once the site of a Roman city, Uricon. He pictures a Roman man, an inhabitant of the town centuries earlier, looking at this same landscape in his day. Housman concludes that the storm, so vicious that it "plies the saplings double," will soon be over, just as the Roman who observed it is now "ashes under Uricon." The thought that many days I was standing in the eye of the hurricane was perversely comforting. The worse our situation got, the more demanding the illness was, the sooner Don would die—or at least have to go to a nursing home—and I could have my life back. The idea that human suffering is universal was also comforting.

My faith also helped. But none of these things, not love or poetry or faith or the fact that Don appreciated what I was doing, ever felt like enough. Every day, the time spent getting him to work and getting him to bed seemed to increase in little increments. Equipment maintenance and failures meant unplanned trips to repair shops and extra work. When I was facing a deadline, and he called from work and needed to be picked up and his pants changed, and I raged and wept as I drove him home because I felt my life was being sacrificed, and I could never finish anything I started, I asked myself why I stayed. The next day might be smooth, but another day inevitably came when the same question arose, demanding an answer: If it's too hard, why are you still here? To my frustration, I never had a definitive answer. Every day I pushed the same rock up the mountain, and every night it rolled back down. Until the day he died, the empty freeway looked tempting. No matter how noble or expedient my reasons had sounded the day before, I never settled the question.

Why we stay in marriages that seem intolerable to outsiders—and frequently to us as well—is highly personal. Barbara Beachman has a theory about why she got sucked into a situation that nearly killed her. "When you put across this persona that you're so strong to everybody, that 'I can do it,' then people let you do it," she says.

When she married Chuck in 1970, they blended families—her four children and his three. Three years later they had two surprises: another baby and Chuck's MS. He was able to work for another thirteen years, but in 1986 he retired and Barbara became his full-time caregiver. Chuck's helplessness would have been burden enough, but the diabetes he developed on top of it, and the fact that the MS caused him constant pain, turned Barbara's life into a free fall toward disaster. She worked the graveyard shift for a local utility company, but when she got home at 7:00 A.M., her day as a caregiver was just beginning. Barbara's voice takes on a singsong quality as she recites a deadening litany of duties. "If I didn't feel like doing any of these things, that was too bad," she says. "It had to be done."

Money problems compounded the situation. With only one income, hers, money was tight, and she still had a thirteen-year-old son, Thomas, at home who needed to be clothed and fed. Social Security disability paid for a home health aide to bathe Chuck twice a week, but that was it as far as home health care. The Beachmans' medical insurance company had gone bankrupt, leaving them with tens of thousands of dollars of medical debt, and even though Barbara had a bankruptcy court document saying she wasn't responsible for the bills, it didn't keep creditors from calling, or the debt from blackening her credit record.

Struggling to keep up with the demands of illness, she found herself more and more isolated. The Chuck she had known, who had loved her children as his own, accompanied her to church, and never missed a Little League game, became angry and demanding. He was mad at God, mad at her, mad at the world. He never thanked her or praised her for anything. Their children, except for Thomas, had moved out, and rarely visited, unable to face their father's decline.

Exhausted, with no possibility of relief, she often found herself in tears. "I was so tired I could hardly get one hand above the other," she says. "I told Chuck, you can't treat me like this. I can't do this anymore." One morning she showered at work, then came home and threw a suitcase in the back of her car. She drove to a nearby park and pulled up under some trees. "There was no 'last straw,'" she says. "I just knew if I went home I would die."

For a week, she lived in the car, going to work early so she could shower there, and using the public restroom to brush her teeth and change clothes. She kept an ice chest with cold drinks in the car, and ate fast food. Although she notified the Visiting Nurse Association that her husband was alone, she knew that by California law she could be charged with abandoning a disabled person. But she was past caring. In spite of her cramped quarters, she was sleeping well for the first time in years.

After a week, the car's engine burned out and she had to go home. Chuck, though chastened, didn't understand why she had left. She wasn't sure, in his condition, that he was capable of understanding. Convinced at last that something had to change, she arranged to take in a boarder, who, in exchange for board and room and a small stipend, helped her care for Chuck. The Visiting Nurse Association, finally awake to the seriousness of her situation, also agreed to donate one morning a week, and Barbara began to get some sleep. She also found a counselor who asked her a question she had never asked herself. "What do you need for yourself?" Barbara could only stare. "It was the most shocking question anyone had ever asked me," she says. "I couldn't answer. All I did was stammer. D . . . d . . . d . . . duh."

With the counselor prodding her to think about her own needs, Barbara began to consider moving Chuck to a nursing home. She met with angry resistance, not just from Chuck, but from their children, who knew she had lived in her car for a week. "Obviously there was something wrong with me, some defect in my character, that I couldn't do all that for Chuck," she says. Her family wasn't prepared for the new Barbara that began to emerge. "I alienated everyone for a while," she recalls. "This was when I started getting strong, but I guess when you've been walked on for so long, everyone considers it bitchiness." It took her two years to do, she sees now, what should have been done much earlier. Now that Chuck is in a nursing home, she allows herself to go to the beach with friends sometimes instead of visiting her husband. He is still abusive and controlling, but she says she will never leave him. "I just don't think I could ever leave him or divorce him," she says. "When I married him, my first husband had just left me and I had all these kids, with no child support, nothing. Chuck worked hard, and every cent went into the house. He didn't drink, gamble, or cheat on me. He helped raise the kids and he was a good provider. I felt I sort of owed him." Her job offers excellent health insurance, and Chuck would lose those benefits if they divorced. She feels "on hold" now, but because it's such an improvement over her caregiving days, she can handle the uncertainty. The new Barbara has a saying pinned to the mirror in her bedroom: "Strong is lonely." She says thoughtfully, "You like to think you're in control, that you're self-sufficient, self-reliant . . . that you're an adult. To admit I'd lost control of everything, that was the hardest step of all."

Some believe their partners would die without the care they provide, and stay because they don't want a death on their conscience. In a more positive light, Bill Hill keeps Peggy at home because he promised her. Even though she is totally incapacitated, he gets satisfaction from having her with him. "Her doctor says that the only reason she's alive now is because of the care she gets. So that's fine. It's very, very satisfying," he says. His determination to care for her at home is all the more remarkable because he doesn't believe she would do the same for him, even though she was trained as a nurse. "She would be too frustrated at the lack of progress," he says.

Love, money, obligation, children—these are some of the reasons partners stay. Often it's a combination of reasons. Sometimes, it's nothing specific we can name that keeps us showing up day after day; as Bette Allbright says, it's just "something that's in us."

A wife's decision to stay is often based at least partly on economics. Even if a husband can't work anymore, disability or retirement pay is often more than a woman can earn. When Don had to stop driving, he was surprised that I began to drive him back and forth to work without complaining. I was surprised he was surprised. Even if I had been able to step into a tenure-track position at a college in Helena, which I couldn't, I knew there was no way, at least for many years, I could earn as much as he was, with his years in the insurance business. It only made sense to keep helping him earn a paycheck. Carly, whose husband, Mike, is awaiting a lung transplant, says, "Mike has a couple of big life insurance policies." Then she considers. "I don't think that's the number one reason I stay," she says. "When he dies, I'll know I've done the right thing. I guess that's what it is."

Most of us want to "do the right thing." We want to honor our wedding vows, to provide our children with a good example, to be respected by our neighbors and friends. We see our wedding vows as a promise we made, not just to our partners, but to the world.

For those with strong religious convictions, wedding vows are a promise to God as well as society. Bill Hill says, "I made a promise to her, and God had witnessed it." Hilde's strict Catholic upbringing allowed her no indecision as to whether Hank, now like another child, was still her husband. A lawyer she consulted about finances advised her to get a divorce. "I was offended," she says. "But then I thought, he's just laying out the options for me." To her, they were unacceptable options. "I just could not do that, in front of the children. I made these vows for better or worse." Donna Keefe was shocked when she talked to other families at the local veterans hospital. "They couldn't believe I hung around," she says. "I guess a lot of wives leave. I couldn't understand that concept. I said, 'Well, where do they go when they leave?'" She insists that it never entered her mind to leave after Pat's unrelenting back pain was diagnosed as pancreatitis. "That was my husband," she declares firmly. Don Crawford says of his wife, Pam, "I wanted to stand by her no matter what happened. I had made a vow to Pam, in sickness and in health. And we had this little girl we were committed to raising."

Children can be strong motivators to stay in a marriage. In any marriage, the arrival of children calls for a reassessment of life-styles, as we ask ourselves whether we want to continue old habits in front of impressionable eyes. Don and I, casual about church attendance before, began going regularly after the children had been baptized. I've written of my strong temptation to run away after he was diagnosed. But every time I indulged in one of my fantasies of packing the car and fleeing to a place of only healthy people, my daughter's little face peered up at me. "Where's Daddy?" she'd ask. I couldn't imagine what I would say. That we couldn't stay with Daddy because he was sick? Could I really say that to my child? Like Hilde, I couldn't abandon my husband "in front of the children." I couldn't model for them that running out on a sick partner was acceptable. I couldn't imagine the precise ways my cowardice would blight their lives, but I knew it would. I would never be able to justify an act so fundamentally unjustifiable. Don had been an enthusiastic delivery-room dad, at my side when each of them took their first breaths. "Seven pounds, I bet," the doctor said as he laid a flailing Megan on the scale. "No, eight," said Don, the fly-fisherman. She was eight pounds, two ounces. He held her before I did, wiping blood and mucus from her face. The idea of taking my four-year-old daughter and eighteen-month-old son away from their father, who adored them, and now had been stricken with a terrible illness, wrung my heart. He might be limited physically, but he could still be a devoted father. And, less altruistically, I needed his help raising them.

Some partners don't think much about why they stay, and the question catches them unaware. They've been swept downstream by a swelling torrent of duties, and find themselves adrift, out of sight of the shore. For them, a numbing depression takes over and makes them feel powerless to choose. They feel that no matter how bad their lives are, at least the pain is familiar. Leaving is full of uncertainty, because there's always a possibility, though it may be hard to imagine, that they could end up worse off than they are. As one woman said, "Fear was a factor in keeping me in the marriage. Where would I go? What would I do?" Most of us, unless the situation becomes truly unbearable, choose the devil we know over the devil we don't.

With the expectations of spouses, children, and neighbors pressing in on us from outside, we have to create some breathing room for ourselves. Otherwise, as Barbara Beachman discovered, we start to die. We realize, consciously or not, that if we're going to stay, we have to find ways to cope. Norma Imber, whose husband, Robert, is in a nursing home, runs two support groups for well spouses. She's developed a theory. "There are two kinds of well spouses. One kind, they're overwhelmed. They're expected to learn nursing home techniques. The nurses give them an hour or two crash course, where these nurses have been trained for one or two years or more. They expect this husband or wife to learn this quickly. Then the spouses go home, and there they are, faced with this very sick person. They learn it and do it, and get into this rhythm of taking care of someone twenty-four hours a day, and they're beating themselves to death."

And then there's the second group. "Some will say, I can't do this. I don't want to do this, and I'm not going to do this. Somehow or other, they will find another way." She doesn't believe either type of spouse has made the "right" decision—but some are healthier than others. "At this point, I've heard it all, and my heart goes out to these people."

Norma believes that some well spouses are able to "find the door." One of her "doors" has been being able to laugh, and making those who attend her groups laugh too—a gift she didn't know she had. "You need to laugh, because if you don't, you sink deeper and deeper, and it's very hard to climb back out," she says.

Dorothea has a part-time job doing genealogical research. The fact that all the people she researches are dead, and safely beyond change, provides a welcome retreat from life as a well spouse. She theorizes that her work allows her to stay with her husband by providing an oasis from the constant ups and downs of his kidney disease. Work, part-time or full-time, provides an area of our lives where we feel valued, gives us something to think about besides the illness, and helps offset the thanklessness of caregiving. Kas Enger says, "I love my job as a secretary. It fulfills me. It uses a lot of my gifts and talents, and I feel very appreciated in the job, and very confident."

Finding the door begins with the realization that we have to take care of ourselves because our partners don't want to or can't anymore. One woman says that her job is important not only for the income it brings, but so that she has another role in her life. After work, she disappears into a back room for an hour. Her family knows she is not to be disturbed during that time, even for the phone. She sips a beer, reads the newspaper, or just thinks her own thoughts until she has to emerge and be a caregiver again. Diane Maxwell takes her hour before work every morning. She lights candles, sits in a recliner, covers herself with a hand-made quilt, and reads the Bible, praying and meditating and gathering her thoughts before the day starts. Although she still sleeps with her husband, Kas Enger remodeled her son's room after he moved out to get married, and created a space that was hers alone. She says, "Now I have a quiet place where I can go and be by myself." Some spouses have affairs, as much for the freedom of being with a healthy person as for the sex.

Nursing home placement can sound like the door, and certainly it eases the caregiving burdens. But it doesn't answer the question, "Why stay?" In fact, for me, the question became harder to answer, because my husband was living elsewhere. It began to cross my mind that if I was going to live alone anyway, why not divorce? But like some others in this chapter, my wedding vows were important to me. I had loved my husband when I said them, and I loved him now. Divorce, after all we'd been through together, seemed like giving up. And there were my children, teenagers now, who might be more negatively affected by divorce than they had been by the illness. After all, the illness wasn't a choice; divorce was.

I signed up to take a writing class at a local college, which would help update my résumé, and I began querying the universities about work as an adjunct professor. I also began to take riding lessons, and allowed myself to dream of owning a horse someday. Joining a support group helped me begin to create a support network that eased me through the last years of his illness and his death. Such groups can become like family because of the life experiences members share.

Listing the changes I made is easy now, but making them was slow and difficult. I worried about the costs, both in terms of money and time. Would these new activities take time that I should have been spending with Don? His comment that I didn't belong in the support group filled me with guilt and doubt. Trying to decide what I owed him and what I owed myself was one of the biggest challenges of his illness. Marriage made us one flesh; if he couldn't do something, how could I do it without him?

Everything hurt at first. Summer evenings, from horseback, I watched the sun set on the purple Elkhorns and cried. I felt like I was mourning for both of us: for myself, because I didn't have him with me, and for him, for all the little joys that he would never experience. Being free to do what I pleased, while he was helpless in his tiny box of a room at the nursing home, seemed the worst kind of betrayal. I felt complicit in the rotten hand fate had dealt him. What right did I have doing things he would have loved to do, but couldn't? For that matter, what right did I have to be walking around on two healthy legs when he couldn't move? The MS had taken so much from him, left him so impoverished, I was terrified that I might be taking from him, too. Through counseling, and time, I came to understand the paradox that giving to myself helped me give to him. I learned to forgive myself for my good health, and for wanting to enjoy it. I learned how to make room for myself within my marriage, and by building in some contentment, I was able to honor my wedding vows. Because I felt happier, I was a better wife to Don, more present, more interesting, more fulfilled. Around that time, I came upon this passage in a book entitled *The Tentative Pregnancy* by Barbara Rothman. The speaker is a woman in her eighties:

> When I had diphtheria, my mother could comfort me, she stayed in my bed with me, she held me—but she couldn't have it for me.

She continues:

> One life to a customer, one to a customer. You're alone. Ultimately we're all alone, we're each alone.

When we marry, we believe we'll never be alone again. That illusion can take a lifetime to relinquish.

As I've said earlier, I also had an affair, which unexpectedly deepened the love I felt for Don.

For most of us, the love we felt as healthy people undergoes a change during illness. Some spouses spoke of loving a partner, but said they were no longer "in love," or felt the same passion they had when they first married. A woman whose husband has had diabetes for eighteen years says, "When you're taking care of all his needs, it's hard to continue to think of him with that passionate love you had at one time. I would go to the ends of the earth for him, but it's just not the same." This is one area in which spousal caregivers are different from other family caregivers. A mother can love a sick child with the same intensity as she loves a well one, and a child can love a sick parent as much as a healthy one, but most of us find it impossible to feel for our spouses that same romantic attraction we felt when they were healthy. Maybe, as the woman above theorized, it takes on more of a parental nature.

Chronic illness is the refiner's fire, and the question of "why stay?" conceals another question, "what is love?" We remember when love was reciprocal, when doors were held for us, or when kitchens, at the end of a long day, were warm with smells of delicious food. With chronic illness, the well spouse does most of the giving. Chronic illness asks, How much do you love him or her? Then it keeps upping the ante. This much? This much? How much is enough? Does it stop when our partners can't give back, at least not the way we want? Is it still love if, in Shakespeare's phrase, it "alters when it alteration finds"?

The love we feel for our chronically ill partners is full of the painful recognition of our shared mortality. We look at this person we've chosen above all others and say, "This could be me. If the shoe were on the other foot, I'd want him, or her, by my side, loving me no matter what." No one who leaves does it lightly, but only when the circumstances allow no other way out.

Loving someone who is chronically ill takes steely commitment. Donna Keefe says of Pat's frequent surgeries, "It takes a little bit of dying, every time I watch him come out of one of those." When a couple is able to maintain some balance in the relationship—when the sick one can still offer the well one something meaningful—they've accomplished a miracle. The Russells have done that. Jim Russell says that, despite the shock and anger Hannah's MS brought, he didn't think about leaving her—and still doesn't. "I loved her no matter what her physical capabilities were," he says. "She's a wonderful person, very special. She has a maturity, a presence of mind."

Though difficult to achieve, loving someone's essential self, regardless of what they can do, is true love. Everything works against us culturally, because Americans put so much emphasis on doing, as opposed to being. Continuing to love under these circumstances is a staggering test of character. Eugenia Staerker says, "Ray would do the same for me, I know he would, absolutely, without a doubt, I know because of the way he acts toward me. He never takes anything for granted, and never orders me to do anything. He always asks."

Barbara Drucker stays because of love, too. "David needs me, he loves me, and while it's not always easy to love him because he's put me in second place to his illness, we have a shared history." She stays in her thirty-year marriage because she'd rather be with David than anyone else. "So that must be love, right? It's not a romantic kind of love. There's no sex life, at least not a satisfactory one to me, but I'd really rather be with him than anyone I know."

Mark Johannes acknowledges the tragic duality of loving someone with a chronic illness. "My life with Bonnie today is in many ways a two-edged sword. We have learned so much about each other, and our love has grown so much in the past twenty-five years." His voice quavers. "I love her too much to walk away from her. And God forbid I ever do, but if I ever do, it'll be because I can't stand to see the pain anymore."

# 10. Partings:
## Our Paths Diverge

Paths diverge during illness, sometimes permanently. Chronic illness is a series of little deaths, over months, over years, that prepare us for the big ones. The big changes take a number of forms: divorce or separation; nursing home placement; and the ultimate one, death. When we look ahead to one of these, it's with a mixture of dread and longing. Although we may believe these partings will allow us the freedom we've yearned for so long, they also bring new problems. As one man said wisely of his wife's twenty-five-year illness, "As for the future, I have learned that it is best neither to fear or want the future too much. The future will take care of itself."

Partners who divorce feel they've done everything possible to save the marriage, but finally come to the conclusion that, whatever else they owe this person they married, they don't owe them their lives. "There's not a right choice or a wrong choice," sighs Steve Kambich, who divorced his wife, Wendy, who has MS. "You go and do what you have to do, but there's not a right and there's not a wrong." They had been married three weeks when Wendy's first symptoms appeared. Advised not to get pregnant by her doctors, who feared pregnancy would worsen her symptoms, she conceived twice on birth control pills. Although she went into complete remission during her pregnancies, after the babies were born, the MS came back with a vengeance. She had such a rapid course that by the time their second child was two, she couldn't walk or control her bladder or bowels. She had so little upper body strength that once, left alone to watch television, she slumped over and nearly suffocated. Despite the help of Wendy's mother, and Steve's mother and sister, and additional home health care, caring for Wendy at home was a struggle. Steve had fallen in love with her happy-go-lucky personality, but her increasing helplessness, especially when it came to mothering her children, made her frustrated and constantly angry. A glass of spilled milk was enough to trigger a screaming fit.

Bankrupt from her medical care, lonely, overwhelmed, and only twenty-six years old, Steve nevertheless tried to stay in his marriage. "I'm Catholic, and I did a lot of counseling with the clergy, and they said no, stick it out, hang in there, and I said OK, I really think I can do that." But, in regard to his sexual needs, he says, "They'd say, 'Well, that's just part of it.' I wanted to say, 'Yes, but at my age, your urges are a lot stronger.'" Still, he'd leave the rectory determined to be a good husband and father.

He was amazed when Wendy's parents suggested divorce. "They said, 'You guys never did stand a chance. You never did get a marriage,'" he remembers. "We'd like to see you get on with your life and meet someone else." Steve was full of doubts. "I guess you could say we didn't get the shot we wanted at this life, but I still didn't feel free to divorce." He loved Wendy, and wanted her to go to a nursing home in their hometown, where he and the children could visit. Her parents wanted to take her to their town, ten hours away. A tug-of-war arose over the best place for her to live. If they were taking care of her, her parents wanted power of attorney, which was impossible if she and Steve were still married. Convinced at last that the burden of caring for Wendy would be done by people who loved her, Steve gave in. Wendy's parents took her back to their town, and Steve kept the kids and filed for divorce. Guilt-ridden and afraid of the emotions it would stir up, both for Wendy and for himself, Steve hasn't seen her for thirteen years, although the children see her at least once a year. He says, "Sometimes I don't think I did a good thing."

Roy Layton's decision to divorce his wife was, for him, a matter of survival. His wife, Donna, had been ill for sixteen years when he was involved in a serious motorcycle accident. He lost one leg below the knee, and underwent two operations on his skull. Donna's demands, combined with his own arduous rehabilitation, led to what he describes as a "spiritual breakdown." "I've always been a person that felt you should keep your commitments, and that your word should be valid," he says. His accident forced him to reexamine those beliefs. He divorced Donna in 1994, but continued to care for her at home for another nine months, when she entered a nursing home. He doesn't feel guilty about the divorce, because he feels he did everything he could for her. He still visits her twice a week. "She wanted me to dedicate myself to her care. Realistically, if I had, she would have totally devoured me with her needs. There would have been nothing left of me."

"I feel we tried everything we possibly could," says Rhoda of her struggle to keep her family together following her husband's stroke. He was forty-four and she thirty-nine and pregnant with their second son when his secretary called her and told her John had been rushed to a hospital. Her husband, a public relations officer, worked hard at getting back on his feet and returning to work. When the baby was born, Rhoda allowed herself to hope that, despite John's physical disabilities, they could be a normal family again. Then John's company fired him. It was the beginning of the end, according to Rhoda. "He said to me, 'I'm never going to work again. I'm just going to wait for the disability checks to arrive in the mail,'" she says. He stayed in bed all day, refusing to bathe, shave, or change clothes. The couple consulted psychiatrists and psychologists, and John tried antidepressants, all to no avail. In counseling, he would agree to help his wife, who was working several part-time jobs in addition to caring for him, but he wouldn't follow through.

More than the lack of support for herself, Rhoda worried about the example he was showing their sons. "I often felt, how can I have these kids around someone who looked and smelled like someone living on the street?" One day, eight years after John's stroke, Rhoda realized she wasn't willing to continue this life. "Here I was," she says, "forty-something years old, celibate, unhappy, married but not married, and I knew I couldn't go on for years and years. I just didn't want to live this way anymore." She ran into an old neighbor and was shocked to hear herself say, "We're probably going to get a divorce." She had never before said the "D" word.

She and her husband have been separated for fourteen months and will eventually divorce. "I don't feel guilty," she says wearily, "because I feel like I did everything I could do." It took her years to understand that John's ability to converse intelligently concealed serious cognitive deficiencies. She says, "Even though he had significant brain damage, none of the neurologists was ever able to say, this is because of that. I guess it's because they don't know."

Don Crawford was shocked when his wife, Pam, urged him to

divorce her so he could get on with his life. "She didn't seem too coherent, so I didn't know if it was just a fantasy," he says. When she repeated her wishes to a lawyer, he was convinced. At the court appearance, "The judge said, 'Mr. Crawford, you're now divorced. Go and have a peaceful life.'" He says, "It was like a benediction. Thank God I was sitting down. Pam's lawyer finally said, 'It's over,' and I said, 'I don't think I can stand up.'" Despite the divorce, he says that he "still feels married" to Pam, and although he has moved across the country, he still visits her in the nursing home several times a year.

As I've said earlier, some couples are forced to divorce so that the sick spouse is poor enough to qualify for Medicaid. The divorce doesn't end the devotion they feel for each other, however. In another ironic situation, a husband recovered from his chronic illness, but is so accustomed to being taken care of, his long-suffering wife is considering divorce. "My support group says life is too short," she says. "But actually, life is too long. People are living so much longer." She doesn't want to spend the rest of her life mothering her husband.

Putting a young husband or wife in a nursing home is a wrenching decision. We know that nursing homes are places where people go to die, not get nursed back to health. There's nothing homelike about them either. Putting a young person into one of these places, where he or she will have very few peers, is especially difficult. As one woman whose husband has had several strokes says, "The very best and cleanest nursing home is wretched." An aging population will come up with more palatable alternatives to these brutal places, and already, smaller "residential homes," which care for fewer people, and offer a homier setting, are springing up. I also heard of a group of disabled people who started a co-op, by renting an accessible apartment building and hiring several live-in caregivers whom they share. Making home health care more convenient, reliable, and affordable could ease the caregiving burdens and keep people in their homes longer.

Because we know that those who check into nursing homes don't check out, we may put the decision off far too long, telling ourselves, against all reason, that we can do it alone, or that things will get better. Maybe subconsciously we're waiting for the inevitable crisis to take the decision out of our hands. And it will come. Barbara Beachman says, "We all wait much longer than we should. I don't know anybody that hasn't. And that's sad."

As in so many areas of our lives, well spouses confront the tyranny of societal expectations in this matter too. We're made to feel that caring for a spouse at home is our responsibility. Maybe we, too, believe that our wedding vows commit us to caring for a husband or wife ourselves. No matter how herculean the task, if we can't do it, we blame ourselves. We've been told all along how strong we are, and may have come to believe it ourselves. Our churches, our families, our friends—all seem to have an opinion about this most personal decision. Even though we know a spouse would be better cared for, and safer, in a nursing home, summoning the "tough love" this step requires is difficult. A nursing home may be better for us and for them, but actually making the move is another matter. Jim Russell says, "More often than not, the stories I hear in my support group are about abusive relationships. It's terrible. I would never put up with that. If I were in an abusive relationship, I'd say, bingo, you're going to a nursing home. But that's not the case here at all." He is well aware that if something happens to him, Hannah will have no choice about whether to go to a nursing home. Still, he sighs, "It's never easy."

We may find ourselves setting deadlines. For some, it may be when the partner no longer recognizes them. For others, it may be when the spouse becomes violent. Some insurance plans, ours was one of them, won't pay for home health care, but will cover a skilled nursing home, so the decision is partly financial. For some, the kids are suffering from too many demands, or being emotionally abused by the sick spouse. Or maybe the sick person's needs have become overwhelming. They've become dangerous to themselves and others.

John Hardin has been determined to keep his wife, Nancy, at home in spite of her increasing mental deterioration, but after nine years is considering a nursing home. One spring day he left Nancy in the car while he took groceries into the house, and she drove into several tables of plants he was growing to sell in his nursery. "It was a big mess," he says. The plants were destroyed and the car was damaged. She also is starting to wet the bed at night. Despite the constant vigilance she requires, John hates to think about this change. "I wish I could put my agony into words," he says. "She has a right to continue living in her own home. But for the first time, I am starting to think about my own rights and needs. She has lost almost all memory. She doesn't recognize any of our friends anymore. She's forgotten our grandkids' names. I still cry about the loss of my wife."

For Catherine Petrina, leaving her husband, Robert, with Parkinson's dementia, in a nursing home has been a torturous in-again, out-again process. Because she missed him so much, she'd bring him home repeatedly, only to have him "freeze up," or begin hallucinating. One night he slipped out and wandered the neighborhood till daylight. She was befuddled, then horrified, when he knocked on the front door that morning, because she thought he was asleep in his bed. Recently Catherine had a stroke following surgery, and she believes it was God speaking to her, telling her she'd done enough. But it had taken a message from God himself to convince her.

Sometimes a nursing home is a matter of life and death, as it was for Debbie Lang. Her husband's dangerous behavior had the family so terrorized they had no alternative. Intellectually, Debbie knows this; still, she is filled with guilt that she couldn't keep him home, and still longs to have him there. Well spouses learn that doing the right thing doesn't necessarily feel right.

Some can be fairly matter-of-fact about the process. Bob Keller says of his wife, Ellen, "She finally got incontinent, and I couldn't handle it." The decision was a little easier because he found a nursing home he liked. He had worked as an inspector for HUD, and had seen many that repulsed him. "That was one thing that impressed me probably more than anything else about the home she's in, that it didn't smell like a nursing home." He put in an application, and was surprised when they called him only three weeks later. "I said, 'Well, it's going to happen anyway, it might as well happen now.'" He missed Ellen, but, he says, "I'm not too emotional, crying and things like that. I did more fishing. I fished and fished and fished."

Sometimes the well partner's own failing health makes a nursing home a necessity. Margy Kleinerman had a mild heart attack, which she believes was stress-related, after her husband, Joe, was diagnosed with Alzheimer's. She has also coped with rheumatoid arthritis for many years. One day her husband sat down at the table for lunch and couldn't get up again. "I made up my mind on the way to the hospital in the ambulance that I couldn't bring him back home," she says. Her three grown children supported her choice. "My oldest son said, 'You have to do it, Mom. We can't have two sick parents.'"

Paul Kleffner's children felt the same way. His wife, Thelma, had a series of small strokes, and her behavior became so erratic that he had to watch her day and night. When his doctor warned him that his blood pressure was high enough to cause a stroke, his children persuaded him to put their mother in a nursing home.

He says, "I cried an awful lot that first year. I couldn't talk about it without crying. There's nothing worse than coming back to the house in the evening and it's just like you left it. It's the hardest thing for me." The ranch he and Thelma raised their seven children on has been declared a historic site, and he has begun a second career giving tours, which has helped him adjust to his new life. A spry eighty years old, he says, "If she were to die, I might consider remarriage, but as long as she's alive, she's my wife."

Pam Cook, a certified nurse's aide, has cared for her husband, Don, at home for three years, and loves her caregiving role. But now her health is starting to worry her. "I've been going for lots of tests," she says. "The bottom line is stress. They can't pinpoint anything. I just regret that I can't keep strong enough to keep doing his care." She is sad and confused. Her sister tells her that her health problems may be a sign that it's time to put him in a nursing home. Don has "a million dollar smile," she says, but it shines as brightly on everyone else as on her. She admits she can't tell whether he appreciates her care, or even knows her. But that makes no difference to her. "If I put him in a nursing home, will I say, 'Sorry, I had to give up on you'? That's how it's feeling, it feels like giving up."

For Linda Anderson, the nursing home decision was eased by their doctor's observation that "hospitals don't do death well, but nursing homes do." She says, "I wanted Steve in a place where they're not fighting you every step of the way. And the people there were wonderful." Still, moving him was the hardest thing she'd ever done. "I remember leaning up against the wall of the bathroom and sobbing until I thought my insides would fall out."

The summer of 1988 was a year of decision for us. For the previous ten years Don's decline had been gradual, but that summer he slipped dramatically. In the spring he was asked to resign from his job as an insurance underwriter, and he was grief-stricken at having to leave a job he loved. Even nature seemed to be conspiring against us, because it was a blisteringly hot, dry summer. The smoke from the fires in Yellowstone Park, dense even as far north as Helena, made me feel like I had stumbled into some kind of hell, and my eyes stung continuously from grief and smoke.

That summer we crossed an invisible line. Don couldn't hold his head up anymore, and even with a new headframe for his wheelchair, the kids and I were constantly lifting his head from his chest. We had so many home health aides coming and going, I told Don we needed a revolving door. I had been willing to move a mattress into a walk-in closet in order to get some sleep at night, and do everything else he had needed over the years, but I wouldn't ask my children, eleven and fourteen, to hold their father's head up for him. That seemed beyond what any family should have to do.

Now that he wasn't working an eight-hour day, he needed twenty-four-hour care. The elaborate "feeding machine" we had bought was so complicated, it was easier to hand-feed him. I told Don I didn't want the kids turned into miniature home health aides. "What about these two children we've brought into the world?" I asked. "They deserve to be kids." I wanted so much to keep him home, but home had to be a place where we could all live—not just Don. At that point, we didn't know if our insurance would cover a nursing home, however. I began to make desperate phone calls to nursing homes, government agencies, and our insurance company. Don told me to stop. "Tell me what else to do then," I said heatedly. "What other options do we have?" Our home was too small to have an aide living in full-time—even if we could afford it. I was often struck by so much craziness coming from something neither of us wanted. The world had been turned on end.

It took an intense family counseling session in our living

room, which I realized later was really an intervention, to convince Don the time had come. I explained that I wanted to keep him home, I hated to think of him going to one of those places, but his care was too hard. I had damaged the cartilage in my shoulder lifting him on and off the toilet, and my back was starting to complain too. "What would have to happen to Chris in order for you to go to a nursing home?" one of the counselors asked him. He started to cry. Then we all cried. I thought I had never been through anything sadder.

Knowing that Dr. Shepard would have to do the paperwork, I laid my case before him, again with that odd feeling of dissonance: Why is this woman pleading for something she doesn't want? He was reluctant. "People don't come out of those places," he said. He hadn't examined Don for a while, however, and was willing to reserve judgment until I brought him in. When he saw Don, he seemed shocked at the changes of the past few months, and didn't hesitate to sign the admission papers. When I suggested that, considering how fast Don was progressing, hospice should be involved now, he agreed. He told me privately he didn't think Don would live another six months.

That evening I got him ready for bed as usual, following our lengthy routine. Don sat patiently in his wheelchair beside the bed, waiting for me to slide the transfer board underneath him and pull him up and over the bed's wooden frame. I looked down at his wasted arms, his sunken chest, his useless legs. I seldom saw them, concentrating instead on the task in front of me. I put my arms around him. "Don't go," I wept. "I can't stand it that you have to leave." If only he could stay and his body could go. It was the MS that was taking him away. He was still Don. He was still the man I loved. I wanted to explain that it wasn't him I was pushing away, only his obstreperous body. "It's as if we've all been walking along the same path, and now the path splits off in different directions," I told him. "You have to go one way, and we have to go another. We can't follow where you're going. And you can't come with us." Then I cried because my love hadn't been enough to save him.

The nursing home we found was as pleasant as those places can be, and he had a private room. On a gray September day we left him there, snow already on the hills, and went home feeling both sad and relieved that now his care was someone else's responsibility.

I knew that continuing to care for him at home was endangering his safety and mine, and the children's psychological health. As a relative said to me later, "Some jobs can't be done at home. This was one of them." Like Debbie Lang, I knew these things in my head, but my heart wanted him with me. Looking back, I think I grieved him more deeply after he went to the nursing home than after his death. By the time he died, he had been gone from home for five years; his death just made the separation final. As a friend said to me about her mother, "I didn't mind her death, but I hated her dying."

Some partners find that, although their spouses are out of the house, they spend almost as much time at the nursing home as they did caregiving. A partner who has been tyrannical at home can be equally demanding from a nursing home, maybe more so, because now he can manipulate his spouse's guilt. Barbara Beachman had to learn to live again after Chuck went to a nursing home. "For so many years, I felt like I had no control over my life. It's a whole new set of skills." It took a year of a counselor "harping at me, asking, 'What do you do for yourself?' that got me to change. I thought it was impossible." Tentatively, she started doing things with a woman friend, and joined a codependency support group. "I didn't realize I was so codependent until I started reading the material. But it really described me to a 'T.'

There I was in black and white." Eventually, she was able to say yes to friends who wanted her to join them, instead of visiting Chuck. She was even able to go to a Fourth of July picnic and take short vacations without him. "That was hard," she says, "because he expected me to do those things with him. So to juggle both of our needs was a challenge, but I started doing it."

Each of us has to find our own comfort level with nursing home visits. Some, and I was one of them, find it difficult to go at all, and want nothing to do with teas, barbecues, or any activities that are not "required." I was furious that Don had to be there, and my attitude with the staff was usually confrontational. After he died, I realized that some of the employees genuinely loved him, and I regretted my anger. Other well spouses find involvement brings peace of mind, and may be helped by attending support groups offered by the facility. Norma Imber spends much of her week at Robert's nursing home. "Since I became a volunteer, they're wonderful to my husband," she says. "I got some extra perks for him, and that's very good too, because when I know that he's well taken care of, then I'm comfortable." As Norma has discovered, patients who are visited more get better care.

The question of how to live as a "married widow or widower" may become more pressing now that we have energy and time for new relationships. The solutions, as I've discussed, are different for everyone. Putting a husband or wife in a nursing home is another in the string of "ambiguous losses" chronic illness brings. Our person is still alive, but can't participate much in our lives. We may wonder how often to bring them home, or whether to bring them home at all if they resist going back, and how to keep them involved in our children's lives. Cutting them out of family life too soon, I believe, cheats them, and us. At first, when he came home on Sundays, Don acted as if his role was that of disciplinarian, and I reminded him that if the kids saw him as an enforcer, they wouldn't look forward to his visits much. I also tried to make sure he got to Meg's high school plays and Tim's soccer games. We had to learn how to recombine harmoniously with our new living arrangements, which took time.

Sometimes relationships actually improve. One woman said that after she put her husband in a nursing home, she dreaded her six-year-old son's reaction. But when she told him, he replied, "Good. Now you won't be so mad all the time."

Nursing home placement forces us to confront a partner's death because end-of-life decisions must be discussed and put on paper. However, the subject may have come up, in a different way, much earlier. One man told me how his wife begged him to leave a loaded pistol on the nightstand one night as he left the house. The request shocked him. He thought about the legal ramifications, but his wife's pleading eyes told him she meant what she said. Finally he decided to put the pistol on a closet shelf. He told her that if she really wanted to get it, she would have to figure out a way. He came home to find her asleep on the floor. He saw that she had tried to knock the pistol off the shelf, but hadn't been able to. Seeing how it troubled him, however, she never made such a request again. "There are times I've wished I had left it out for her," he says. "For the simple fact that I've seen what she's gone through."

Margo Brooke had mixed feelings when she discovered her husband's body in their fume-filled garage. She had thought that his ALS had progressed to the point that he was incapable of arranging his suicide, and realized she had been wrong. "I wasn't angry that he hadn't told me he was planning it," she says, "because then I would have had to be part of it. And I wouldn't have wanted that. I don't think it would have been fair to my children, either." She wasn't angry at him for taking his life. "It's like abortion," she says. "I wouldn't do it, but I think others should have the option, and I hadn't walked in his shoes."

Most of us would probably avoid talking about end-of-life decisions indefinitely, but nursing home placement forces us to. Deciding what kinds of medical procedures should be used if a person can't breathe or swallow can cause conflict, but at least you're forced to talk about them. Barbara Beachman's husband has been resuscitated seven times in the nursing home. "It makes me angry, because with the kind of life he's living, why he wants this so badly, I do not understand," she says. Because Don went into the nursing home as a hospice patient, and hospice nursing is restricted to "care and comfort only" (in other words, no heroic measures or treatments), our options were more defined. Still, the fact that he wanted antibiotics to treat infections was frustrating for me. I had to respect the fact that, as sick as he was, these choices were his to make, not mine. But as I've said earlier, after a certain number of near misses, I learned not to immediately go into "crisis mode," gathering the children and calling relatives, every time he ran a temperature. So his choices helped me make mine. Having the guidance of hospice counselors helped us find the riches in his dying. Our society is so bent on seeing death as the enemy, we don't see that dying, like so many other aspects of chronic illness, brings opportunities as well as obstacles. The kids and I had a chance to say four last things: I'm sorry, I forgive you, I love you, good-bye. These honest exchanges would have been impossible if we had been fighting the reality of his impending death, and I believe they speeded our healing.

Fran Oswald had been paralyzed for four years when he began telling Pat he was ready to die. "We worked through everything," Pat says. "We had long conversations in the nursing home, hours. We talked about how much we loved each other, and if we had done anything to hurt each other in sixteen years of marriage, we forgave each other. We reminisced about our fun times, and our disappointments." As Fran requested, Pat mixed his ashes with those of his beloved schnauzer, Whiskers, who had died earlier in Fran's illness, and scattered them in the backyard. Because they had talked out everything, Pat says she has "no guilt. None. Zero."

One Sunday in January 1993, I broke Don's hip while transferring him from his wheelchair to the bed. No one had warned me that his hip bones were fragile as old china after so many years in a wheelchair. I was simultaneously stricken and relieved that I had been the one to do it, knowing that one of the aides would have suffered terrible guilt. Dr. Shepard advised Don to let it heal on its own, but he was in pain, and wanted hip replacement surgery. I was baffled and furious. With his whole body disintegrating, I argued, why replace one part? The operation, long and grueling, seemed like gratuitous agony after all he had suffered. After he went back to the nursing home, I had to stay away. None of his decisions was making sense. When, a few weeks later, he developed a post-op pneumonia, I still couldn't believe he might be dying. He had nearly choked to death on many occasions, and in the past two years had had several bladder infections, one so bad the previous summer I called his brothers and sister, who came for what they thought was a last visit.

So, in spite of all the signs, I almost missed his death. When it came, on a Sunday morning in February, Tim and I were by his side, and Meg had called from college a few minutes earlier. The most difficult thing to see was his labored breathing, which left him unable to talk. Then, as Tim and I held him, his eyes rolled back and he took a couple of ragged breaths. His jaw came up as though he might say one last thing, but changed his mind. Then he was gone. That he had died so peacefully after so many years of struggle, and that I had been there to see it, was a last gift he had given me, one I didn't feel I deserved. His death had the same numinous quality as the moments we shared in the delivery room, after each of the children was born.

My immediate feeling was one of relief. At last it was over, for him and for me. I didn't have to witness any longer the humiliation of this man I loved so much. Joan Fanti, like most well spouses, knows this feeling too. Her husband, John, was quadriplegic from a broken neck for seven years. A few months after he died, she watched a movie about a woman whose son had AIDS and had come home to die. She says, "And she looks at him after he's died and she says, 'It's better for you, and it's better for me.' And when she said that, I fell apart. I thought, that's right. It's better for him and better for me."

I wasn't sure what to expect from the grief process that lay ahead. I wondered how much grieving I had done already, and how much I still had to do, as though there might be a prescribed amount written down somewhere, figured according to body weight or some other formula. In spite of the work of Kubler-Ross and others, grief remains a mysterious process. While certain aspects vary from person to person, some seem to be universal. I still went through the numbness stage, even though his death had been so long anticipated. I know, because I don't remember much about his funeral—none of the people who were there—and my sister tells me that on the phone the day he died, I "sounded like a robot." I began to come out of that the day a weeping fig tree was delivered as a condolence gift, and I started to cry when I remembered how Don had loved them, and had wanted me to get one for the living room. Why hadn't I? I berated myself. Why hadn't I visited him every day, cooked his favorite foods more often, been more patient? Why had he been cheated out of a life, this good man who had spent most of it mired in illness? I grieved the life he had never had.

My anger, at least, was gone. Maybe because I had so much of that emotion during his life, it had burned itself out. A few months before he died, Don told me, "I'm not mad at anybody or anything," and maybe the level of peace he had achieved helped me set aside my own hurts.

No matter how much we anticipate a death, grief eludes pre-planning. No two people share the same personality or background or previous grief experiences. Each of us grieves a unique individual, and a unique relationship with that person. Describing "stages of grief" implies that people move through them in order, at specified times. If we're not at a certain stage after three months or three years, we wonder if something is wrong with us. If we're still in pain after the second year, we're afraid we took a wrong turn somewhere. How can we tell if we're normal? For me, someone who has always trusted her head over her heart, learning to trust feelings was a new and uncomfortable experience. During Don's illness, I relied on my head to get me through, for, as one wife said, "How can you fall apart all the time?" Now that he was dead, I had to let go, but didn't know how. I had to bang my head on the fact that grief was an emotional process, not an intellectual one, and was out of my control. Only after I began to think of it as similar to the labor of childbirth, as waves of pain followed by intervals of peace, did I begin to heal. And the birth metaphor is apt. We do give birth to a new self through our grieving.

Well spouses worry initially that they're too relieved, that they should feel more grief-stricken. Linda Anderson said, "I thought I had done a lot of preliminary grieving, but I had a lot to do. I was surprised at the intensity of the pain. I was somewhat pleased, in an odd way, because I thought maybe I felt less for him than I should. So when I went through that grieving, it was almost a comfort to me, that I could still care so much."

Well spouses may have an advantage in that death has been a long time coming, and we have a network of single friends to help us. We may also have begun to think like single people again, and to develop interests and activities of our own. Having these aspects of our lives in place eases the recovery process.

Having been a well spouse marks us forever. One spouse pointed out that it was like a birthmark, something we can never scrub off—no matter how much we want to. We are permanently changed by the experience—and we should be. We have a piercing awareness of the shortness of life, and the uselessness of material things, and we take a new set of values into the life that lies ahead. David Herndon, whose wife Kay's illness took everything they had financially, isn't bitter. A year or so before she died, he took her out on their favorite lake, and she saw a fawn in the woods. "The lake in Tennessee, where I would spend all my free time in great pain, is now a place of gratitude," he says. "We took Kay's ashes and spread them where she saw the fawn." Her illness has had a radical effect on the way he lives now. "You see someone lose everything, and see how little it means, a house, a car, a job," he says reflectively. "I have no interest in those things. I've been changed completely by this experience."

Naturally, the past colors our view of the future. Linda Anderson says, "I did things I never wanted to do, and don't ever want to do them again, thank you very much. I've thought about this, and if I met someone . . . I'd have to have a certified letter from heaven, that he'd never get sick."

Anger is a natural reaction to grief. One wife said, "I gave too much of myself away, and I feel so emotionally drained. I really should remarry within the next five years, because I did like being married. But I've gotta tell you, I feel so turned off on men and on marriage."

Another widow is full of ambivalence about caregiving for her husband, who was critical and demanding, during his kidney disease. "I did everything a good wife was supposed to do, and got left with big insurance policies. That's a good thing," she says. But she admits she is angry, although she is not sure why. After all, she says, "I did everything I could, a real 'Johnny on the job.' Maybe I should have done more for myself."

Now, finally, we're able to grieve fully. Before, we had to grieve our partners one loss at a time. Now that they're dead, we can end the endless cycle we've been stuck in. We forgive ourselves for not being perfect when our husbands or wives were alive; we know we did the best we could in punishing circumstances. Near where Meg and Tim and I scattered Don's ashes, at the base of a towering aspen tree, I hung a bronze marker inscribed with Jesus' words after he summoned Lazarus from the tomb: "Unbind him, and let him go free." For so long, Don had been bound hand and foot by illness. At last he was free. I felt a kind of fierce joy that now he could go wherever he wanted in his changed, and blessed, state.

Maybe we realize we could have done more to take charge of our lives, and we're determined that the future will be different. Shirli Schwabe, whose husband died of scleroderma, says, "Nothing can do a number like sickness. I feel if we can get through this, we can get through anything. I know the life I have ahead of me is going to be what I make it."

# Afterword:
# Finding the Door

 "I try to choose, every day, to make it the best day I can," says one wife. Choosing to find the positive in everything we encounter is the key to well spouse survival. I know I was "lucky"; my husband died after fifteen years. Many well spouses, however, can expect their husbands or wives to live as long as they do, or to outlive them. They can't look to anyone else to save them. They must create their own happiness, making use of whatever and whomever they need to make an unbearable situation bearable.

It is possible, and the well spouses who had adapted best shared certain traits. First, they'd taken responsibility for their own survival. "Go for a walk with yourself," urged a counselor I saw early in Don's illness. Every well spouse needs, first of all, to identify the sources of satisfaction in his or her life, those "pockets of pleasure," as one wife termed them, and devote time to doing those things daily, if possible. Even in the best marriages, we become what our spouses want us to be. Chronic illness calls for a reassessment. Now that they aren't able to do those things with us, do we still want to watch Hitchcock movies or spend Saturdays on the golf course? Maybe not. A spouse's illness means that leisure time becomes precious. Squandering it on activities that don't fulfill you or people who drag you down isn't helpful.

Mentally healthy well spouses have discovered a balance between love and independence. Having identified the things that renew them, they insist on taking time to pursue them, sometimes over the objections of their spouses. They report that getting away regularly, sometimes for several days at a time, is a necessity, and well worth the extra money and planning such escapes require. These spouses tell themselves that, because of their own arduous duties, they and only they have the right to decide how and when they will spend their time. This kind of independence takes self-knowledge, self-love, and courage. Such spouses have come to understand that they can't pour from an empty cup. They've learned to say to their families, friends, and partners, "I understand you don't want me to do that, but I'm going to do it anyway." Then they follow through, with a minimum of guilt, knowing that if they're going to function at all, they must take care of themselves.

They've created lives apart from the illness. They have jobs that make them feel effective, and interests that nurture a self that isn't defined by chronic illness. They don't let hopelessness color every part of their lives. Because they see themselves as more than just caregivers, they're able to model a sense of optimism for their children, and the assurance that life doesn't have to feel constantly out of control.

They have strong support networks. They've assembled counselors, both professional and nonprofessional, friends, family members, and support groups they can depend on to provide emotional sustenance when it seems the sun will never shine again. As a result, they never feel alone, knowing that if they reach out, someone will be there to listen, and to laugh and cry with them.

Last, they've made the experience a spiritual journey, which helps them see beyond their own troubles. While this journey may not have led them to a deity or a specific religion, it has led them to a larger view of the universe, which enables them to put their own woes in perspective. Through their suffering, they've become more aware of the suffering of others, and they've become givers as well as takers. By sharing the wisdom they've gained through hard experience, they're able to forget, for a while, their own trials. They've learned to make their difficulties serve them.

# Where to Find Help

**Alzheimer's Association**
919 North Michigan Avenue, Suite 1000
Chicago, IL 60611-1676
800-621-0379; in Illinois 800-272-3900

**American Cancer Society**
1599 Clifton Road NE
Atlanta, GA 30329
800-227-2345
512-927-5791 FAX
www.cancer.org
E-mail: webmaster@cancer.org

**American Diabetes Association**
1660 Duke Street
Alexandria, VA 22314
703-549-1500
800-232-3472
www.diabetes.org

**American Heart Association**
7272 Greenville Avenue
Dallas, TX 75231
800-242-8721
800-AHAUSA1
www.americanheart.org

**American Lung Association**
1740 Broadway
New York, NY 10019-4374
212-315-8700
800-586-4872
www.lungusa.org
E-mail: info@lungusa.org

**American Paralysis Association**
500 Morris Avenue
Springfield, NJ 07081
800-225-0292
Spinal cord: 800-526-3456
www.apacure.com

**American Parkinson's Disease Association**
1250 Hylan Boulevard
Staten Island, NY 10305
800-223-2732
www.apdaparkinsons.com

**American Stroke Foundation**
96 Inverness Drive East, #1
Englewood, CO 80112-5112
800-749-4152

**The Arthritis Foundation**
1330 West Peachtree Street
Atlanta, GA 30309
404-872-7100

**Chronic Fatigue and Immune
Dysfunction Association**
P.O. Box 220398
Charlotte, NC 28222-0398
800-442-3437

**International Polio Network**
4207 Lindell Boulevard, #110
St. Louis, MO 63108-2915
314-534-0475
314-534-5070 FAX
www.post-polio.org
E-mail: gini_intl@msn.com

**Leukemia Society of America, Inc.**
600 Third Avenue
New York, NY 10016
212-573-8484
800-955-4LSA
www.leukemia.org

**The Lupus Foundation of America, Inc.**
1300 Piccard Drive, #200
Rockville, MD 20850
301-670-9292
800-558-0121
www.lupus.org/lupus

**Myasthenia Gravis Foundation**
222 South Riverside Plaza, #1540
Chicago, IL 60606
312-258-0522
800-541-5454
www.med.unc.edu/mgfa
E-mail: mgfa@aol.com

**National Academy of Elder Law Attorneys, Inc.**
1604 North Country Club Road
Tucson, AZ 85716
520-881-4005
www.naela.org
(This organization cannot refer you to a specific lawyer, but can tell you what questions to ask a lawyer in your state.)

**National Alliance for the Mentally Ill**
200 North Glebe Road, #1015
Arlington, VA 22203
703-524-7600
800-950-6264

**National Association of People with AIDS**
1413 K Street NW, 7th Floor
Washington, DC 20005
202-898-0414
202-898-0435 FAX
www.napwa.org

**National Chronic Fatigue Syndrome and Fibromyalgia Association**
3521 Broadway, Suite 222
Kansas City, MO 64111
816-931-4777

**National Family Caregivers Association**
10605 Concord Street, Suite 501
Kensington, MD 20895-2504
301-942-6430
800-896-3650
www.nfcacares.org

**National Kidney Foundation, Inc.**
30 East 33rd Street
New York, NY 10016
212-889-2210
800-622-9010
www.kidney.org

**National MS Society**
205 East 42nd Street
New York, NY 10017
800-344-4867
www.nmss.org
E-mail:editor@nmss.org

**National Organization for Rare Disorders**
P.O. Box 8923
New Fairfield, CT 06812
203-746-6518
203-746-6481 FAX
800-999-NORD

**Parkinson's Disease Foundation**
710 West 168th Street
New York, NY 10032
212-923-4700
800-457-6676

**Well Spouse Foundation**
610 Lexington Avenue, Suite 814
New York, NY 10022-6005
212-644-1241
800-838-0879
www.wellspouse.org

# Bibliography

Carlton, Lucille. *In Sickness and in Health*. New York: Delacorte, 1996.

Cohen, Marion Deutsche. *Dirty Details: The Days and Nights of a Well Spouse*. Philadelphia: Temple University Press, 1996.

Cole, Harry. *Helpmates: Support in Times of Critical Illness*. Louisville: Westminster/John Knox, 1991.

Drattell, Alan. *The Other Victim: How Caregivers Survive a Loved One's Chronic Illness*. Santa Ana, Calif.: Seven Locks Press, 1996.

Karr, Katherine. *Taking Time for Me: How Caregivers Can Effectively Deal with Stress*. Amherst, N.Y.: Prometheus Books, 1995.

Kroll, Ken, and Erica Levy Klein. *Enabling Romance: A Guide to Love, Sex, and Relationships for the Disabled*. New York: Harmony Books, 1992.

Strong, Maggie. *Mainstay: For the Well Spouse of the Chronically Ill*. Revised and updated edition. Cambridge, Mass.: Bradford Books, 1997.

Welsh, Linda, and Marian Betancourt. *Chronic Illness and the Family: A Guide for Living Every Day*. Holbrook, Mass.: Adams Media Corporation, 1996.

Wolpe, David. *In Speech and in Silence*. New York: Henry Holt, 1992.

Here are two books that can help you discover the benefits of journaling:

Progoff, Ira. *At a Journal Workshop.* Los Angeles: Tarcher/Putnam, 1992.

Rainer, Tristine. *The New Diary.* Los Angeles: Tarcher/Putnam, n.d.

# Index

abusive behavior, 54, 55, 57–58, 124–25, 126–27
accessibility issue, 29–30
adaptive equipment, reluctance to use, 28, 31–33
affairs. *See* extramarital relationships
AIDS, 6, 224
alcohol abuse, 13, 34, 76, 123, 130
Allbright, Bette and Jim, 17, 93, 121, 180, 188
ALS (Lou Gehrig's disease), 6, 113, 146, 210–11
Alzheimer's Association, 221
Alzheimer's disease, 36–37, 41, 58, 111–12, 126
  diagnosis of, 11
ambiguous losses, 20, 64, 209
American Cancer Society, 221
American Diabetes Association, 221
American Heart Association, 222
American Lung Association, 222
American Paralysis Association, 222
American Parkinson's Disease Association, 222
American Stroke Foundation, 222

Anderson, Linda and Steve, 23, 60, 70–71, 120, 128, 170, 176, 205, 214–15
anger, 5, 105–35
  acceptance of, 130
  causes of, 107
  children as targets of, 140–42
  of children of chronic illness, 140, 149–51
  communication and, 57
  counseling for anger control, 134
  dealing with anger, strategies for, 57, 124–26, 129–35, 150
  denial of, 119
  disagreements and, 33–36, 128–29
  at doctors' callousness, 116–18
  evolutionary purpose, 129
  exercise for, 131
  at family members' lack of support, 107–12
  forgiveness and, 107–11, 134–35
  at friends' abandonment of sick person, 107–10, 112–16
  guilt and, 121, 124, 129
  helplessness and, 120

# About the Author

Chris McGonigle is an honors graduate of Mills College and received her Ph.D. in English from the University of Washington. She was a well spouse for fifteen years after her husband, Don, contracted multiple sclerosis. He died in 1993. Her work has appeared in *Woman's Day*, *Family Circle*, and frequently in *Woman's World*. She lives in Montana.